Everything Begins With

ASKING FOR HELP

Everything Begins With

Asking for Help

AN HONEST GUIDE TO DEPRESSION AND ANXIETY, FROM ROCK BOTTOM TO RECOVERY

KEVIN BRADDOCK

An Hachette UK Company
www.hachette.co.uk

First published in Great Britain in 2019 by
Kyle Books, an imprint of Kyle Cathie Ltd
Carmelite House
50 Victoria Embankment
London EC4Y 0DZ
www.kylebooks.co.uk

ISBN: 978 0 85783 676 2

Distributed in the US by Hachette Book Group,
1290 Avenue of the Americas,
4th and 5th Floors, New York, NY 10104

Distributed in Canada by Canadian Manda Group, 664 Annette St.,
Toronto, Ontario, Canada M6S 2C8

Editor: Tara O'Sullivan
Cover design: Kari Brownlie
Typesetting: Paul Palmer-Edwards
Copy editor: Jacqui Lewis
Editorial assistant: Isabel Gonzalez-Prendergast
Production: Caroline Alberti

A Cataloguing in Publication record for this title is available
from the British Library

Printed and bound in the UK.

10 9 8 7 6 5

CONTENTS

TO ANYONE SUFFERING

Thanks for opening these pages.

This is a book about two of the most common mental illnesses (depression and anxiety), where they can lead (breakdown, burnout or crisis) and what happens afterward (recovery).

In this book I write about these things because they're what I know, and I share them because I reckon that what I've learned going from rock bottom to recovery might help. It offers some ideas and guidance, information and anecdote, along with the hope that things will improve. That's all.

Here is an idea of where we'll go. This isn't a set of steps that, followed to the letter, will guarantee a new you or your arrival at a perfect state of got-better-ness. Instead they're a general direction of travel – some things to think about on the way.

1. If you're at rock bottom, you can only go up.

2. Ask for help and keep asking.

3. The body wants to move and doing so helps the mind.

4. Tell your story, honestly.

5. Listen to what people have to say, and learn new ways to live.
   Recovery means anything you learn that helps you feel or function
   better.

6. Back to number 3: keep moving.

7. Hangovers won't help, so stay sober if you can.

8. When smartphones, social media and technology become too
   much, get into the elements. And vice versa.

9. Forget purpose for now. Your life will find one when it needs it.
   Instead make getting better the meaning of your days.

10. Love the people around you, and (this might be harder) let them
    love you.

11. Life is a combination of the things that happen to you and the
    things you do every day. So start building helpful practices every
    morning.

12. Things will change – this is the only guarantee – but there isn't
    "a way" apart from the one you find. So take the time to find it.
    Patience is a virtue.

13. Practise gratitude: when you do, everything looks better.

PART I

ROCK BOTTOM

CHAPTER 1

EVERYTHING BEGINS

How things look when the sun comes up

Days

Can I tell you what mine look like?

Some mornings I wake up and feel okay. Get out of bed, make some coffee, then sit drinking it while reality condenses from the fog of dreams into familiar forms. I roll the blinds up, and listen to the sound of the planes passing way above. I feel okay – yes – the day is okay. Rub my eyes, sit for a while and then get on with daying: the stuff that happens in the day.

Other mornings might bring a few clues that I'm sliding into a depressed phase, and I notice some familiar markers: making simple decisions becomes really tough; my voice goes quiet, and I feel afraid of being heard or saying something wrong; and I get furiously angry about intrusive noise: headphones on the bus, or loud eating noises, rowdy conversations conducted on hands-free.

Still other days I wake up and things seem grey and empty, colourless and hopeless – reason-less. I feel lonely and tired, my body feels slow and heavy. I'll feel as if I've screwed my life up, or my life is screwed up. I repeat the routine above and maybe some energy eventually arises, petering out and then reappearing through the day.

On days like these it's time to do some work so I'll try a combination of:

Walking: out the front door, down the road; stop to tie my shoelaces again; then into the park and round it once, maybe twice.

Speaking: saying a few words under the breath. "I'm just walking around the park, it's Monday" – that kind of thing. Later, I'll ring someone, just to talk and mobilize my voice, remind myself that that's what it is for: to speak.

Stretching: legs, arms, torso, down to the toes, up to the sky, making circles with fingers locked together. Hamstrings and spine. Nothing elaborate.

Moving: remembering my body to my mind, bringing the two back together. Maybe go for a run, practise some intricate tai chi moves.

Listening: to whatever's there. Birdsong, the voice of the wind, those planes. Over in the skatepark, there's a guy playing a trap mixtape on his Bluetooth speaker.

Looking: what colour are the leaves against the white sky this morning? They're darker – dryer – than a few weeks ago. Soon they'll tend toward brown.

Sensing: what am I worried about, this morning – what does that stirring I notice mean? There's always, always something, but as usual these first thoughts are amorphous. In my mind I make a list, trying to contain them in words. I get to number three but then the attention drifts off.

Breathing: that's it – just breathe. I'm sitting on a bench now. Start breathing, because most of the time I forget to do that, apart from the automatic breathing that keeps me alive. Close the eyes, count to 10, 30 or 50 if I have the patience.

Accepting: all I really know, sitting there in the park or back at my flat, is that these phases come and go. Sometimes there's a trigger I can identify, sometimes not. It calms me a little to remember that.

Really simple stuff. The day begins.

And still other days I wake up and just get dressed and get out the door, get on with some work, meet a friend, go to my tai chi class or recovery group, the shop or post office, an event, or just off to hang out and be part of a crowd. Chat, chill and have a laugh. The day may be fantastic or it may be forgettable. Days like this don't need any thinking about.

In the sweep of time most mornings don't feel the way they did five years ago, when I had one wish for these waking moments: not to be depressed. This was what I'd tell people when they asked me what I wanted from life, back then. Just to wake up and not be depressed, nor to feel anxious, because I felt it every morning.

Depression: a hard, flat hopelessness that rendered me silent and static, emptied of all energy, belief, love and joy.

Anxiety: right on waking, an electric current of fright running through me, thoughts like a whip. Panic thoughts turning into panic feelings. Head-in-hands dread.

Every morning, and much of every day.

There's one particular day to talk about here: the day I hit rock bottom, when I couldn't cope any more and tried to end my life (and came close to it) – the day I asked for help. The day when everything changed. We'll come to that soon enough.

Since then the days have passed as I describe above, with gradual improvements over the years, but they've all had one theme in common: recovery, this work of getting better measured in mornings and moods. Doing something every day to get better or stay well or, if neither of these lofty ambitions are within reach, then functioning at least.

Dealing with it, plodding on, finding a way, enjoying things, coping with others, living again.

Us

Recovery is a big word so we can look at that too, but first there's something more urgent to talk about, which is this: why should you trust what I've got to say about dealing with depression and anxiety, and travelling from rock bottom to recovery, which is the path I've been on the last five years?

It's a fair question, and to answer it I'll tell you what I can about myself, the stuff I learned from people I've met and the things I did that helped, along with some things that happened to me.

I'll also make a promise: a promise not to make any other promises. I won't press a programme on you or a series of steps, saying, "Follow me, do this and you're guaranteed to get better, cured or transformed." There'll be no certificate for achieving a "Best Self".

I won't yell solutions at you or demand you sign up for my online course. I won't insult you by offering "empowerment" or "inspiration", things that suggest you're not good enough already, or what you've got to hand isn't sufficient. I can't give you a better you – reformed, cleansed or somehow perfected – and I definitely won't try to make you happy. No therapist worth their chaise longue would ever direct a client to *do something*, and that's another reason I won't (and in any case, can't) tell you what to do.

I won't even argue that there's a cure or an answer for what we know as depression and anxiety – after all, I haven't found one. As my days suggest, these things come and go, like the tide of the sea or cycle of the sun.

Instead I want to talk to you in a way that others talked to me – seriously and honestly – and to do that, I won't be sentimental in this book, manipulating you into feeling pity for me. That won't help either of us. And I won't be comic or ironic either, playing my shortcomings for laughs in a bid to make you like me. That isn't necessary either. Watching comedians often leaves me with the impression that being funny is a performance against sadness, a way of alchemising it into something else, making it palatable. This book is directly about sadness. Reading about depression can also be depressing, so I won't put you through any war stories either, pornographic depictions of the depths of despair.

None of these things seem necessary, but trust does, and perhaps by my telling you what I know this way and filling in some gaps by talking to others, you'll feel some reassurance or hope that recovery is possible. That what you're going through can be got through when you find the path that's yours alone. Or, at the very least, that we can find a way to talk about it.

I'll show you how I found a path and a language, and some of the things you can do to find your own.

So

I'm Kevin: I'm in my mid forties and I'm from a small town in Shropshire, England. I grew up there with my mum and dad (who were teachers) and my sister, and I went to school there. In 1990 I went to live in London, a place I was afraid of, and I did a degree in French at Goldsmiths, University of London. Soon after graduating I started work as a journalist, first for music magazines and later for fashion magazines, writing stories about trends, youth culture and social issues. I've also been a DJ, triathlete, cyclist, consultant, washer-upper, mentor, speaker, publisher and… well, I've done all sorts of things, many of them involving language in one form or other. I speak French fluently, Italian and German conversationally.

In 2009 I went to Berlin for a couple of months and stayed there until 2014. I'm a man: a heterosexual, short (5ft 6in), white, bald, single, no kids. I rent a flat in south London, and friends and family are scattered around the UK and beyond. My mum died at the end of 2017 (cancer), and I was very sad and upset about it.

I wonder what you'll make of these facts, what picture they paint of me. I can't know this, and to tell the truth, it's a bit laborious writing out this life-CV, the parts of my identity as I see them. I'm conscious of an urge to make myself sound successful or interesting, emphasizing my achievements and the cool stuff I've done (interviewing Justin Timberlake or Daft Punk, DJing at parties, working in fashion).

But as I said before, I'll be serious in this book, because putting on a show is something that makes me uncomfortable these days, but in a way it's also what this book is about: the façades we create. And when I say serious, I don't mean being serious because mental illness is a solemn subject. I mean serious about how we relate and how you hear what I say.

Another version of my story is below and maybe it will build this feeling between us, some companionship. It's a sort of psychic CV of my awkward inner stuff that I put together through years of therapy, thinking about stuff, writing things down and going through life. Being up at times and down at others and fluctuating, sometimes severely, between being terrific company and a total misery-guts; searching inside and outward, being angsty, depressed, anti-depressed, cheerful and just okay, like those days I talked about above.

First memory: I'm on a beach in North Wales, playing in a shallow pool of water. My family are walking away from me and I feel like I'm being abandoned (they didn't abandon me, by the way; this is a feeling, contained in a memory).

11 years old: My granddad died, and for the first time I wondered what the point of living was when people you love die or go. Maybe I should die too, I thought. I was in a maths class at the time, in the first year of comprehensive school.

15–16 years old: In school I was good at French and decided to read some books by French philosophers (Jean-Paul Sartre and Albert Camus) who argued that life had no inherent meaning and whatever we do is futile because we're all going to die one day anyway. I hadn't really thought about "the meaning of life" before that, or even if life needed one. Life doesn't need meaning when you're just living it, playing with mates, going to school, watching TV, pursuing hobbies (skateboarding, rock climbing, building dens, books and music were mine). I began to feel this futility, although perhaps I was performing it at the time – sort of miming being depressed, just like I was mimicking the sounds and mannerisms of French as a way of learning to speak it. Still, these depressed Parisian existentialists seemed cool and meaningful: they smoked and drank while talking about deep things, looking good in black and white photographs.

20 years old: I was living in Edinburgh with my two best friends and had a summer job as a washer-upper in a restaurant. One day I noticed something strange in my perception: I felt weirdly removed from reality, as if it, or I, wasn't quite there – like a pane of frosted glass between me and, say, the plates drying on the rack or the chef yelling at me. A tiny, troubling lag between event and perception, like being in a trance. I found out later that this was called "depersonalization".

20 and a half years old: I was due to spend the next year at university in France, but the night before I was to fly out, a friend in a pub in

London suggested we take some magic mushrooms. We thought it was a good idea; actually it was a really dumb idea. I freaked out, didn't sleep all night but somehow got to France and began looking for a place to live. I started having panic attacks, which I thought were flashbacks to the magic mushroom trip: I'd feel this "depersonalization" effect and then, thinking that I was tripping again, I'd start sweating, my heart and thoughts racing. Very soon I was terrified of going mad. I returned to the UK and saw a doctor who diagnosed "stress-related depression" and a psychiatrist who wrote down "obsessive-compulsive disorder". I was put on a course of antidepressants, which slowly ironed out the twists and tangles in my thoughts and feelings. I stayed in the UK for a while and did some voluntary work with the caretaker in the school I went to – painting walls, sweeping corridors, fixing things – then went back to France, finished that year and then finished university. A year or so later I came off the meds and felt okay again, but I found life really terrifying for a while, for much of my twenties in fact. I was "hypervigilant", another word I only learned later.

29 years old: a wave of disruption arrived. I'd been in a relationship for most of my twenties, but my then-girlfriend and I split up. I found a new job and lost it, then started a new relationship but it didn't last, then found a succession of places to live in that I then had to move out of. A period of drinking way too much, staying up far too late, partying much too hard and driving too fast. I bought a scooter, got a tattoo, thrashed myself in the gym and built some pecs and abs, along with the beginnings of a drink problem, and wore expensive Japanese jeans. It lasted a few years and in the middle of it, phasing every day between icy anxiety and the grey fog of depression, with panic attacks and episodes of depersonalization that emerged seemingly from nowhere, I went to see a doctor and poured out my feelings. I did a bit of therapy and was put on antidepressants, and I've been taking them ever since.

You might think that all this would have built some wisdom or caution into me: made me a bit more mindful about how I lived and cared for myself, over these years coloured by depression and anxiety (by the way, the word "mindful" wasn't used much in the 1990s and

2000s). But it didn't really; I just learned to cohabit with these things as they inhabited me. What I mean is that being gloomy or sorrowful, or fretful and preoccupied, became completely normal: it just seemed to be me, the person I was.

However, I did have the wit in my mid thirties to find a therapist to see if they could help with making sense of life. Should all this be normal? And was there a better way: a fuller, perhaps even happier, life? Other people looked quite happy about their lives: I'd seen them. Was it possible for me? Sometimes it was, and quite often, but I knew that waiting out of sight in the hinterlands of consciousness were these ghosts, always ready to reappear.

I carried on living much the same contingent, freelance life for most of my thirties. It may have looked carefree and gadabout but inwardly I felt very lost. Around 2008 I thought I needed a change, so I went to Berlin. At the time I'd been into triathlon racing – swimming, cycling and running – and wanted to run the 26.2 miles of a marathon, so I signed up for the Berlin race and started putting in the long hours and miles of training.

Life assumes gravity in one's thirties; the questions get bigger: money, career, property, pressures. But personally, my rather random life seemed to be getting more random by the year, so I thought I'd embrace the randomness by randomizing it further and going to live in a city where I knew one and a half people.

In the end I lived in Berlin for five years, 2009 to 2014.

42 years old: "Major Depressive Episode" was what the doctor wrote down in my medical record on 10 August 2014. I was in a hospital in the centre of the city, not far from the TV Tower. It was a boiling hot Sunday afternoon and some friends had pulled me up off the pavement outside the office block where I worked and manhandled me into the hospital's crisis centre.

I was a wreck, "a broken man", as they say: mute, drunk, tearful and swamped with panic, dread, shame and confusion, barely able to stand, let alone speak.

They'd come because I'd put a message on Facebook saying, "I need help".

17

I'd posted this message because, somehow, I couldn't use my voice. I'd typed the message out after a few hours sitting there deciding on ways to end my life, running through the list of well-known methods (you'd know the ones I'm talking about, we don't need to repeat them here).

I'd gone into the office and written out a resignation letter to leave the job I knew was gradually destroying me. I'd started crying and then left the office.

I'd gone back down to the ground floor and there was an off-licence nearby, so I decided to drink my way to unreality.

And I was doing it because it seemed like the only thing to do. I'd begun moving toward something that I felt in front of me, around me and inside of me: a void, a vicious blank nothingness, expanding fast.

By ending my life, I could unify myself with it, become one with it, the un-me. Bottles emptied fast, bottle after bottle, reality was dematerializing into a murk. I was on the way but as I was doing it, an alternative thought came, though I don't know where from, and I guess I'll never know.

– I could ask for help. Why not do that?
– *But how?*
– What about Facebook, which you gaze at hour after hour, day after day?
– *But that's not what Facebook is for, no, right? Or is it?*
– Maybe. We can find out.
– *But what should I say?*
– How about "I need help": try that.

I typed those words in, adding my phone number and location, then waited a while because I was wondering whether to post it. What would people think? I was afraid. Maybe they'd laugh or tut, think I was causing a fuss or seeking attention, that I was weird or... well, I don't know what.

I waited for some time, and time passed, I don't know how much. An hour? I don't know, I was just afraid.

I pressed the Post button.

The phone soon went red hot, bleeping, flashing, ringing. Overhead the August sun was blazing, everything was silent. A flock of birds used to swirl around the TV Tower toward the end of every afternoon, but not today. Then friends came in a taxi, scraped me up and took me to hospital and I told the doctor in the clinic what I've just told you here, my whole history as best I remembered it and as best I could explain it. The whole lot.

I could hardly stand but it was the first time I'd ever laid it out, from beginning to end. The doctors asked me to promise that I wouldn't kill myself, so I said the words "I promise".

"Schwer Depressive Episode" is what she wrote down. *Major depressive episode.* From suicidal ideation to intention to action, with an idea and then a reprieve.

What happened after that rock-bottom moment is also what this book is about.

Questions

Reading all this, perhaps you have some urgent questions already:

- Why did you feel that way?
- How had it happened?
- What is this void and nothingness you're on about?
- What do you mean by "unifying yourself" with it?

I can try to answer these questions, but to do so I have to explain something about the gaps in the sequence of "because" in the passage above. I've described the course of that day as best I remember it, but then as now, the further into this moment I go, the more the logic of cause and effect begins to break down, as do language and words. Today as I write this, as back then in the teeth of crisis, things stop being rational and explainable because this is the process where mental illness, something I'd known for a long time, becomes genuine unreason: an absence of all reason and logic, a madness.

To put it another way: when life feels like shit, it may be natural or reasonable to think, "My life is a mess, I hate myself and want to die." A passing everyday thought, one so common that people have written pop songs saying the same thing. But when those thoughts are intense and persistent to the degree of wanting to carry them out – when an idea turns into an intention and then into an act – this is something different. It came on rapidly and aggressively, like the slogan: Just Do It.

I say this because, once again, for you to trust me I need to describe where all this took me and what I saw at the brink I returned from: a precipice overlooking this void and this nothingness, where there is no Why or Because or "here's-the-reason" in any rational, logical, cause-and-effect way that we might understand it. Something that has no form or substance because it is the end of existence: what I glimpsed was the nothingness at the end of what I knew to be my life.

I also mean something situated in time rather than space (the location itself is nothing special: it was a concrete plaza between two office blocks in the middle of Berlin with bike racks, bins and a tramway). So, even if they aren't original or pretty, *void* and *nothingness* are the closest words I can find to describe this moment: a vast, powerful and seductive nothingness that promised an end to everything: to all torment and trouble, the need to take decisions and responsibility, the demand to be me. The destination to which depression beckons, which I moved to meet and embrace.

If it sounds like I am labouring this description, it's because I want to be precise: this is what being a step from suicide looks like, and it's useful to describe, firstly because others have obeyed the call and gone beyond. And secondly because, even if I didn't know it then, this place offers a distinct sign, a placard pointing in one direction.

If we're at rock bottom, we can only go upward. And the great thing about rock bottom is that it's the best foundation for recovery.

Today

Relax. Sit back and breathe.

I'm glad that part's over, said out loud and written down. It took a while to do that, it's one of the heaviest things to talk about. It's never an easy moment to return to.

The events of that day sound extreme compared to the more prosaic drift of panic attacks, depersonalization, OCD, depression, anxiety, self-medication, GP visits and meds that went before it. The crisis moment came on suddenly, but this shift in tempo and intensity seems to be in the nature of crisis as I experienced it and have heard about it happening to others: silently and imperceptibly stuff accumulates over weeks, months and years, suddenly accelerating and leading to something with a range of names: nervous breakdown, burnout, major depressive episode, mental health crisis. Some of these are diagnostic, clinical terms, while others are more colloquial: handy descriptors to provide a simple explanation if anyone asks. The most colloquial of all is "rock bottom" and if we psychoanalyze that a little, it probably means: an admission of desperate need, an inability to cope, final recognition of not being able to carry on and a breach with shame. That's what is was for me, in any case.

It came on fast. Around ten days before I was taken to hospital, one of my staff, Jeni, pulled up a chair next to me in the offices of the magazine where we were working. We chatted for a while and she asked how I was doing. She'd intuited something, and it was the first time anyone had asked me that question for a while.

"Not so good," I said, staring at my shoes. It took a while to identify what exactly wasn't so good, but some elements sharpened into view. The job I was doing – the editor of a fashion magazine – was perpetually stressful. It had been since I started, two and half years before, but, on the whole, I'd managed it. I'd also caught glandular fever (mononucleosis), which added a novel facet of bodily misery – a sort of lifelessness in the muscles – to the terrain I already knew. I was, again, drinking too much. I was also in love but the relationship I was in had hit a tough patch and there were conflicts and arguments I didn't know how to handle. And I was full of doubt, struggling with what to do and how to be: labouring under massive, unanswerable questions every day. It could have been a "midlife crisis" too, had it not also seemed like an extension of the crisis I'd been having since my "quarter-life crisis" at the age of 29.

Jeni listened patiently as I mumbled on and, describing it all, I was surprised at how much content was there. Every day felt like a battle and every morning the questions seemed bigger and deeper. I was still up-right and able until a week or so later when I woke up a with a whirring, needling, all-over anxiety feeling, as if my entire body had toothache. I rang my mum and dad and told them I didn't think I could cope.

The odd thing, looking back, is that all of this seemed normal and ordinary; just my lot, at that particular point in my life. Just get on with it.

The blast radius of mental illness

Ordinary: it's an appropriate word because while common sense suggests this kind of thing shouldn't be ordinary, these days it is. It's far from uncommon to see people going through this gradual then rapid decline, and perhaps you know it yourself. In the last few years it's become evident to me that almost everyone I know has either struggled personally with a mental illness problem (or "issue", to use the American euphemism) or they themselves know someone who is struggling with one, two, or a number of them, wired up in their unique and personal way. Certainly in my life, a number of friends have had breakdowns, been signed off work, sought therapy and treatment, or over the years taken meds and dealt with mental illness, at times successfully and at other times less so. I've seen them fluctuate in and out of being well enough to live and enjoy their lives, and at other times being unable to.

In that same period of time I've also seen how mental health and illness have become much more socially visible, occupying a greater part of the everyday conversation, like (but not, as yet, enough like) something that can be talked about as easily as a broken shoulder or shingles, the natural wear and tear of living.

We often read of celebrities suffering dramatic breakdowns and going into rehab, and hear of people at work having burnouts and disappearing for six months or a year. And often – way too often – we hear reports of the people who stepped beyond the void I gazed into and didn't make it back. In 2018 alone, there were the high-profile deaths of the chef Anthony Bourdain, the designer Kate Spade and the DJ Avicii. Mental illness, burnout, breakdown, suicide: these are as much features of life in the celebrity-media stratosphere as sex scandals and awards ceremonies.

There are also plenty of equally famous statistics relating to all this, which you probably know: the figure suggesting that one in four of us will suffer a mental health problem in any given year; the other one saying suicide is the leading killer of men under the age of 45 in the UK.

Looking at suicide specifically, there are some signs of change, including positive ones. In 2018 the Office for National Statistics reported that the suicide rate for men was at its lowest (15.5 per 100,000) since they began keeping records. There were 5,821 suicides in the UK in 2017, with men making up three quarters (4,382) of that figure. The global average for suicides has been dropping for the last 20 years.[1] In the US, however, the rate is up by 18 per cent since 2000 and a recent report in *The Economist* newspaper highlighted three other critical groups: young women in China and India, middle-aged men in Russia and older people everywhere are more likely to kill themselves.[2]

In the UK there was also news from the National Health Service (NHS) that, compared with a decade ago, ten times as many girls under 18 in the UK are admitted to hospital for a substance overdose, while admissions for self-harm in the same group have doubled in 20 years.[3]

In one way, I don't find these stories surprising even if they are saddening: on the contrary, they seem like evidence of the collateral damage involved in living in the twenty-first century, which is complex, maddening and mapless. They also give the lie to one of the big myths that we labour under: the "Cosmic Should" of happiness, which suggests that we should all feel gratified and fulfilled, all the time. It's a strange idea when you think about it in historical terms: personally, at least, I think of happiness as a fleeting, evanescent thing that usually evaporates the moment I try to capture it.

No doubt these stories and stats raise the profile of illnesses such as depression and anxiety, keeping them on the news agenda, but they also do something else, which is to obscure the stories of low-profile suicides and the everyday experience of being depressed on the train to work or experiencing anxiety while sitting at the desk: where mental illness is a real, lived, experienced thing.

For example, it hit me hard when I heard about the death of a man I met in 2018. Gareth was 41 and a member of an arts project in the town where I grew up. I met him when I went to this arts project to deliver a talk about my own experiences. After the talk we chatted for a while about running, diagnoses, sobriety, meds, and we exchanged emails and stayed in contact. He said that for some time he'd lived with bipolar disorder, and had had times of dealing with it well, and other times of struggling severely.

A few months later, a report in the local newspaper talked of a man who'd gone missing. I looked at the photo and identified the guy I'd met in the room above a shop. Several days later another report said that Gareth's body had been found. Some weeks later still, I went back up there from London and met with Jo, who ran the arts project, and she told me how lost and devastated everyone in the "blast radius" of Gareth's death was. The shockwaves of "Why?" radiated out from his suicide and when they reached me, I felt a sharp sense of meaninglessness too. I was at a birthday party in London when I'd heard the news, and I was upset. That evening, I made my excuses, got a cab, went home and thought about him.

This is what I mean when I say this knot of ugly material – depression, anxiety, breakdown, suicide – is ordinary: something you hear about almost every week. The "blast radius" phrase above was coined by the American academic Lawrence Lessig, who was talking about the effect of his friend's suicide, and it captures the impact of such an event very well: blast radius refers to the distance from the centre of detonation, everything contained in it that will be affected (or "impacted"), and the event itself.[4]

We could also talk about the "mental illness radius", by which I mean that most of us have either had some problems ourselves, or know someone who is suffering.

Of course, it's impossible to tell whether these days there's genuinely more mental illness around or simply more talk of it: more stories told, books written, reports broadcast and confessions delivered, more technologies built to deal with it and greater efforts to dismantle the stigma that surrounds it.

What is genuinely new is the breadth of openness to talking about all of this, and a clue to its extent lies in the fact that the subject spans two different planes. There's the media virtual plane of news, memes, tweets and sensation where famous people are suffering or dying, and then there's the plane that you and I inhabit: the realm of the everyday with its hearsay and rumour, the conversations held in offices and trains, over the phone or down the pub. The story you heard about that friend of a friend who'd been having problems.

Media reflects life and offers a sensation of it, but can't ever capture it completely. On the other hand, sorrowful news that arrives through word of mouth or a telephone call does something else: it creates a feeling of proximity, something mortal, literally closer to the bone and in that sense more truthful – an honest reminder of what we can be, which is fragile, limited and prone to crisis even if most of the time we're totally fine. It reminds us that mental illness is not just ordinary but close and real, and not simply some abstract drama unfolding on a screen. Ordinary stories from the everyday sphere shift the experience from the sensational and the sentimental to the real and the actual. And I say that because I've lived with a foot in each sphere, the mediated and the real, and I've seen the difficulty in talking about it and dealing with it from both sides.

But for all that, I want to talk in this book about four things in particular, because they're the ones I know: depression, anxiety, breakdown and recovery – what they mean to me, how I've navigated them and what I've seen and heard that's worth passing on. These are also big words with fluid, shifting meanings, so to describe their contours I'll tell stories about what they've meant to me and find out more from others who really know, adding anecdotes together to cement everything into shape.

Again, I want to be precise so that you hear clearly what I offer, which is that maybe you'll be able to relate to or identify with, or draw from the ordinary reality of living and dealing with mental illness that can't be conveyed by stats or stories teleported down from the celebrity stratosphere.

Thinking about the self in "myself"

Actually I try not to think of it too much, but when I do, I think of myself as a writer: someone who authors narratives on the subjects above and publishes them (I mean, makes them public) in different forms – printed objects, packs of playing cards, YouTube videos, Instagram posts – with two particular messages. The first is "Ask For Help", which, in that critical, gazing-into-the-void moment, could for someone mean the difference between dying and surviving, recovering and moving on. I believe in this message because, of course, it's what kept me alive, and I'm glad it did. But I also believe it's valuable beyond and outside of that moment.

The second is more of a principle than a message, and it's about practice: the idea that life is a combination of the things that happen to you, and the things you do every day: habits you cultivate, the routines you keep, the stuff you practise to get well or stay well.

Occasionally I think of myself as a storyteller, even if it's a rather ostentatious title (it was given to me by the person who employed me at the last job I had). Nevertheless, it seems to fit because over the last few years I've told this story of how I hit rock bottom, asked for help and began on the path to recovery, which is an ongoing process rather than a single event in time. I wanted to put this story out in the world to say that there's a way forward, no matter how dark and hard things seem in the depths of mental illness.

In 2017 I presented this story in the form of something called *Torchlight: A Publication About Asking for Help*, which is a magazine I made with my friend Enver Hadzijaj, who lives in Berlin. Enver is a designer and artist, and he was the person who came to pick me up after I put that message on Facebook. Allow me to explain why I wanted to say all this stuff.

I was outpatiented at the clinic in Berlin after being taken there in August 2014. The doctors had said that there were a range of wards I could go into, but that the depression ward was full at the moment; it would make sense for me to be an outpatient and call in regularly to see the doctors. So I went back to my flat. My mood was fractious and volatile at the time: I felt cornered, confused and afraid, shockwaves of anxiety coursing through me followed by bleak and silent moods, and an overwhelming sense of exhaustion. Getting from the chair to the table in the living room was a massive effort.

This exhaustion was a result, I reckon, of finally "letting go" – in other words, admitting I needed help, setting down the burden of life and finally allowing others to help me. Like an extreme version of what often happens when we go off on holiday: suddenly able to relax after the prolonged stress of work and everyday life, the body and mind respond by going into repair mode, and as a result you often feel worse, while the beach, the bar and the tourist attractions beckon.

So I'd lie in bed trying to get my head round what had just happened: was this what "a breakdown" was like? I'd heard about others having one, but it didn't seem real. But then, nothing seemed real.

I'd get up and sit on the floor for a while, drinking coffee, then need to lie down again. Scribbled some words down in my notebook, and looked out of the window. Any contemplation of the future instantly filled me with dread; it was all too much.

During these first few days friends were coming up to my flat and checking in on me, to see how I was, and if I needed anything, to talk or open up or just hang out. I was really touched by their concern, particularly because none of them seemed to be fazed by the truth of what I was at that point: a mess, basically. This episode had been quite public, plastered all over my otherwise carefully curated Facebook page. So, I could hardly pretend that everything was okay. Meanwhile, all those Facebook friends whose disapproval I was so afraid of – and this was really surprising to me – seemed to be okay with it too, adding messages such as "you are loved" and "stay strong". One friend had launched a campaign to fill the newsfeed up with pictures showing me in happier times, stuff we'd done together and places we'd been. This feeling of being cared about blew me away.

One message really got through to me. A guy I hadn't seen for at least a decade was messaging me every day, asking how I was, what I was doing and so on. Then one day he offered a suggestion: "From now on Kev," he wrote, "you need to be completely honest and open about all this stuff. Confront it all head on. And seeing as you're a writer, why don't you write it all down?"

This seemed like good advice. After all, I'd spent years either avoiding or ignoring the uncomfortable inner truth that I'd struggled with depression and anxiety; or in conversation euphemizing it and covering it up, or creating a cool or comic persona to distract attention from how I actually felt. It had also never occurred to me that my own life could be a subject worthy of putting pen to paper for.

I wondered why my friend was so insistent on this strategy.

"It's because my sister had what you're going through," he replied, one day. "And she didn't make it. She took her own life."

I didn't need much convincing after that. I started keeping a journal of thoughts, feelings, memories and dreams, along with collecting photographs and making childlike word paintings with watercolours. I kept it up for the next few months as I moved back to the UK, and over the next two years carried on scratching down sentences, longer passages, memories, lists and helpful things I'd heard, filling up Moleskine notebooks and Post-it notes. Eventually Enver and I gathered everything, sorted it through and put it together into *Torchlight*. What you're reading here is an expanded version of that story, perhaps more reflective and less urgent, more dippable-into, with actionable stuff to help if you're going through something similar.

As I hope is evident now, asking for help has been an important thing in my life: a pivotal point when everything changed. There's more I'd like to share about this, but there's something more urgent to deal with, which is about language and the words we use to talk about this subject, beginning with a question: what exactly are Depression and Anxiety anyway?

How we talk when we talk about mental health

I thought a lot about that in the time that followed the crisis.

A couple of months after being taken to hospital, I moved back to the UK to live with my mum and dad in Shropshire; my family wanted me around while I was beginning to recover. Deposited back in the town where I grew up, I found myself with no job, money, routine or purpose other than to begin dealing with this *major depressive episode*. In the end it took two years to write the text we eventually published as *Torchlight*, and it was an exercise in making sense of what had been happening to me – a kind of self-help therapy in understanding and ordering experience through writing, along with finding a way of talking about it that, I hoped, would make sense to other people, and maybe even reflect some of their own experiences. Offer something to identify with.

I realized that to tell this story I needed a new way of saying things, explaining myself. As a professional writer I've been used to modulating my tone of voice to tell stories to different audiences: a register that works for a story in the *Financial Times* wouldn't be appropriate for an avant-garde German fashion magazine, for example. This was the creative challenge, but it was also a distilled version of a much longer-term process in my life, which was to do with explaining or presenting myself and the way I felt honestly and, in doing so, overcoming the intense shame I'd long felt about being who I was: the guy who'd been editor of a glamorous fashion mag, who got scraped up off the pavement and taken to a crisis centre. For a long time before this episode – for most of my adult life, in fact – I'd felt myself to be somehow just not good enough: lacking, needy, unlovable and filled with doubts, conflicts and torment. I've often thought that depression *is* shame: the feeling of simply not being good enough.

Then I remembered what my friend had told me: confront it all head-on, be completely honest and open. So, I thought, I'll just say all this as directly as I can. Copies of *Torchlight* arrived back from the printers and, slowly, over weeks and months, people began to tell me what they thought of it. One friend said it made him very sad and happy at the same time. One guy I know said it saved his life. And once it was published, people who had read it began to write to me. One such message said "Suffice to say your story is my story; along with hundreds, thousands or (probably) millions of others... and yes, it helps."

It seemed that people responded to this way of saying stuff, above all, and it took a while to find this voice – a language that lets others in – and it's the same one I'm using here, to talk to you. A manner that I hope is plain but friendly; I'm thinking about how you hear what I say, guessing that you feel the urge to judge me, but that you might also identify. Things I say may resonate with you and articulate something familiar. At the same time, I don't want to decorate or poeticize what I say, nor blind you with science or jargon. In any case, I'm not an expert on anything apart from my own experiences and even then, only insofar as I know them.

The other reason for speaking this way is that if we're to treat depression and anxiety as common problems, and show that reaching a point of rock bottom is not some exotic phenomenon but an eventuality that seems to happen to people indiscriminately, then to explain and understand it we need a language that's just as ordinary or human, which situates these experiences in the lives we live, instead of in clinical manuals.

At present we don't really have one. In fact, the language we're given can actively obstruct doing so. There's plenty of terminology and defini-tions: the clinical-diagnostic vernacular of "episodes" and "disorders", the convenient acronyms and the universal categories of "mental health" and "mental illness" and, increasingly, nebulous notions such as "wellness", "well-being" and even the new concept of "mental fitness" (which to me sounds a bit like something out of a propaganda film from the totalitarian era). But we might also ask in the first place whether mental health is a thing in itself, or simply the absence of mental illness, which is what this book is about: dealing with something difficult.

Some of these terms seem like straightforward analogues to their physical counterparts, where we're either "well" or "ill"; but it's rarely so simple when they're mapped onto the infinitely more complex terrain of thought and emotions. These terms can be useful, and detailed explanations and codifications can be found online or in DSM-5, the *Diagnostic and Statistical Manual of Mental Disorders*, which is published by the American Psychiatric Association, or the ICD10 (International Classification of Disease), the manual used in the UK and much of Western Europe. Back in our everyday non-clinical world, "depression" and "anxiety" are signal words that help us find a way into this massive topic and the near-infinite breadth of the human experience by saying, "Here, this is what I'm talking about, this enduring misery, this acute fright, and not conjunctivitis or the price of stamps."

However, this language still lacks the nuance that really helps us understand what we're dealing with and, more importantly, to convey it. It may be stating the obvious to say that we need to start talking about (what we call) mental health and illness, if only because in the UK at least for so long we haven't. But what I mean is that we can only deal with (what we call) depression and (what's known as) anxiety by addressing them in the first place: recognizing the shadow in the mirror, admitting it and describing the effect of it, what it means for us.

This isn't to say that depression and anxiety don't exist. They do, they can be lethal, and I'll keep using these words in this book, even if often they function no more effectively than emojis: fixing meaning but doing so a bit too rigidly, perhaps too conveniently or cutely.

But if it sounds like I'm a stickler for words, it's because in writing and speaking I've wrestled with language so that it doesn't imprison me in meanings that aren't my own. I've also been fortunate to work with a therapist who gently steered me away from the emptiness of clinical words, and helped me see the subtleties between depression and despair, or anxiety and feeling afraid, the shades of grey and graduations between them. We've worked together for a while now, and doing so has helped me understand myself, and generate a vocabulary to describe what I've felt and thought during those years.

Stories

There's one more dimension to this language question I want to talk about, which is this: recovery as we're talking about it in this book begins with wanting it to happen (asking for help), and what comes next is speaking about it. We speak in stories.

Words build sentences and sentences build stories, and stories can capture experiences – and conveying experience can help connect us to others. This is important because mental illness isolates people, and the cruellest trick it plays is to convince the sufferer that they're alone. But in telling stories one to another, you to me and vice versa, we're no longer alone, and by giving voice to experiences we're no longer hiding them.

Storytelling is another uncertain word but here I mean it as a way to dismantle shame by explaining who and how you are, extracting your story from the locker of personal, internal experience and using it to navigate the world. Another way of looking at this is that when you've suffered with mental illness, or you've had a diagnosis or a disorder, then you automatically have a story too: something with ups and downs, twists and turns, ins and outs. You may feel, as I have often done, that mental illness has stripped you of your identity, ambitions and everything except your pain. But that already sounds like the opening line to a story that's yours alone.

So here is the first suggestion in this book: start writing your story today, and return to it as you read through the chapters. Make a habit of noting things down with a pen and paper, or make a voice recording or use the video camera on your phone. I'll offer some more ideas for adding to it as we go on.

Meanwhile, despite looking for one in the last few years, I've yet to read a really good manual about mental health and illness, and that might be to do with what we've already said: that unlike, say, the flu or a broken leg, everyone's version of depression and anxiety is their own, hence it's impossible to offer a one-story-fits-all solution. But this also means that, considered in a certain light, all the greatest stories are mental health and illness stories because they capture something of the trouble and complexity of human life, with its arcs of success and failure, confusion, loss and redemption: Hamlet and his existential dread, the sense of life's absurdity described in *The Outsider* by Albert Camus; the deep solitude in Hemingway's *The Old Man and the Sea* and the blur between fantasy and reality in *Alice's Adventures in Wonderland* by Lewis Carroll. None of these stories are headlined as mental health or illness stories, but perhaps that says more about the narrowness of the terms themselves.

Stories tell the truth in the way that statistics rarely do, so if you're in the middle of something, it probably has a beginning and an ending too: the three things that every story needs.

This story

Stories help to contain experiences. The chapters in this book are grouped by subject rather than presented in chronological order, as stories commonly are, and the ideas and experiences I talk about are based on what I've known and learned in the last few years as the events, fevers, sorrows and joys of my life have also developed, shifting around in time and space, accelerating at times and slowing at others. I've kept on writing and speaking, and doing so has helped me see a story – a shape in time – and with it, some learning and meaning in periods of often severe disruption.

However, I need to qualify something from the passage above, which is that there hasn't really been an ending, or not in the Hollywood sense at any rate, with a final moment of hugging and understanding where the actors turn to face the gorgeous sunset, and everything is resolved: completed, answered and done. Outside the pages of this book, my life has gone on in a "to be continued…" way with delights and despairs but the material I include here is written from a position of a-bit-betterness: better as in functioning, relatively stable and able to look at events with some distance and say, "Okay, that happened, this is what I found out, here's how I felt I changed." And perhaps qualitatively better too: I feel like I'm a nicer person these days, or at the very least kinder and a bit less impatient.

I hope it doesn't cause any extra worry if I add that like stories, recovery may never end: there's no cure for depression and anxiety. On the other hand, because recovery does happen and when it's done well it involves a significant change in a person's life, it may prove so powerful an experience that they may never want the process – the story – to end. The drum and bass artist Goldie put this better than I can. I interviewed him a few years ago and he was talking about how getting into yoga helped him recover from a crippling addiction: "I've learned so much from the mistakes I've made that I'm thinking about making a few more," he told me.

One mistake I made was lacking any faith or trust that things would turn out okay, and that I'd be able to deal with the problems I had and handle what life threw my way. So while we're talking story, here's one more anecdote.

Soon after asking for help and being taken to hospital, probably when I was back at my flat trying to make sense of what had just happened, I heard of a useful visualization, something to try out (I'd probably read it in a book, or seen it online). It went like this: if you're going through a really tough patch, imagine yourself from five years in the future returning to your today-self with a message. What message would your today-self want to hear? In my flat I thought about it for a while, and guessed that the best I could wish for was that things would eventually be "alright".

Today, as I write this, I'm that five-years-ahead-me, and I can see that in the intervening years, with their ups and downs and ins and out, things really are "alright". The basic sequence of events that were nailed onto the canvas of reality in those five years looks like this:

In 2013 I was in Berlin, somewhat lost and panicked, with an obscure sense that something in my life needed to change. I'd been there a few years by that point, having moved from London in 2009, and much of what went before remains blank in memory. Nothing seemed to mean very much.

Then, 2014 was the rock bottom year. It started well: I'd quit drinking, and felt cheerier and more optimistic. I was in love and rediscovered a love for life itself. Suddenly things began to collapse – illness, stress, overwhelm and the return of some old and familiar adversaries, anxiety and depression – but I hadn't spotted the warnings. In the autumn I returned to the UK for a while to get my head back together, then went back to Berlin, then returned to the UK once again, this time for the foreseeable, at the end of November.

I spent the winter living with my parents: a cold, desperate and dislocated time when I helplessly wondered what I could do to improve my state and help my situation. Scribbling things down, reading books, trying things out: body hacks, philosophical ideas, creative practices – anything that offered a toehold.

In 2015 the heavy weather began to shift and a friend offered me a room in his house in Bristol, so I moved down and carried on working on the things that seemed to help. Later that year I found a job in London and was semi-homeless for a while before finding a place to live. I went to work and wrote things down, and signed up for a university course. One day I met a lady on a train – we'll come to this – and the pamphlet she gave me made me realize I needed to do something with this vague story I'd been writing.

Nothing eventful happened in 2016, but disruption comes like the weather: early in 2017 my friend Enver and I finished making our *Torchlight* publication and put it out, and by the end of the year we'd sold out of everything we printed and I'd appeared on the cover of a national magazine, left my job and been with my family as my mum died; bedside in the hospice in November, holding her hand as life drained from her.

It's 2018 as I write this, and this path of recovery continues; the story goes on. Writing these passages is the latest chapter.

It's been "alright" in the sense that against every terrified belief I held, I've coped; got through it; got better, lived, learned and begun to like life again. And my guess is that you will too.

* * *

Perhaps we're getting ahead of ourselves here, a bit lost in abstract ideas. But briefly, I need to repeat something: in this book we're not trying to be happy, because happiness isn't the opposite of depression or anxiety. We're looking for a way through the worst and upward from rock bottom, into recovery, with the assurance that there is a way.

Writing and telling stories is one way to do that, so I'll tell you a few more of mine in the hope that they'll help you. It certainly helps me to know that they might. But before all of that, something important needs to happen.

CHAPTER 2

VOICE

*Asking for help, along with thoughts on crisis, shame
and honesty rather than vulnerability. Plus why depression isn't just
"A Man Thing" even if it wounds men in an especially cruel way*

Everything begins with asking for help

So why don't we do it? After all, it's quite simple: you open your mouth and say to someone, "I need help" or "can you help me?". A straightforward, honest request.

Here are a few possible reasons we don't do it:

- Because people might laugh

- They might judge

- You'll feel weak, because you show that you need something

- You might appear (ugh) needy

- If it's to do with mental health, you don't ask because you think you haven't got the "right kind" of problem

- Or a problem that isn't severe enough

- Also, you don't want to bother people

- Or you want to protect them from some difficult inner secret: once it's out, it might cause chaos

- You can't admit to yourself that you need help

And lastly:

- You don't ask because you don't know that there's a problem

Suddenly it doesn't look so simple. Truth is, asking for help is never easy because admitting need can make people feel ashamed. Even in mundane situations, with a tricky piece of work, say, or a decision to be made, it's no easy thing because to ask is to expose a weakness: after all, we're meant to be independent, autonomous and somehow need-less these days, certain of what we're doing and the way we're doing it. There's also the fear that if you do ask, no one will be willing or able to help anyway.

To speak is to enter the world beyond your skin, making yourself real, known and heard – but shame silences, and shame is what stands behind those reasons above. Let's stay with the deadly conjunction of shame and silence because it can, indeed, prove deadly: at least, it almost did in my case five years ago, slumped outside a Berlin tower block, with a failure in the motors of speaking.

Words

As I guess you've noticed, I'm writing this as a man – a man talking about feelings, often volcanically uncontrollable ones. Feelings may often be considered feminine things, but they're universal, spanning the genders. In the last chapter I talked about the awkwardness of mental health language with its disorders and acronyms, terminology that makes our experiences sound like objects in a laboratory. I also talked about the value of stories, but something comes before all this: I mean words, which carry the grain and variation in states of feeling.

Asking for help needs a vocabulary, and talking about this subject of suffering and getting better is, first and foremost, about finding words for it. And by the way, you don't need to be a professional writer to do it; in fact it's probably easier if you aren't one.

To put it another way, the vernacular we've inherited to talk about depression and anxiety masks something else: a deeper idiom that carries the nuances of emotional weather.

When I think about the shades of grey stirred into my own version of depression, there's:

Sadness: it's a reaction to bad news, or the lingering of guilt; the sorry-for-someone-or-something feeling; the response to a situation where I could have done more or better.

Melancholy: which is bittersweet. A memory infused with delight and disappointment, which is bearable when I roll it around my mind.

Sorrow: when I'm up against a hard truth; someone has gone or something been lost, and neither will return. Here is where tears begin.

Misery: a response to lasting painful circumstances beyond my control: an awful situation at work, dreadful weather, tense and endless waiting.

Despair: a defeated feeling, as if a tragic instant has been stretched out into a perpetual moment (usually, nothing actually tragic has happened; this is a psychic event, existing in my mind).

(What I call) Depression: it's flat and hard, a prolonged despair that seems to bend the laws of time, making it seem eternal and unending. Neither feeling nor numbness, more the impossibility of all feeling – living-deadness. This is where it becomes physical, too: there's exhaustion and the engines of moving, speaking, feeling and doing grind to a halt. This is when I'll start telling people "I'm depressed".

And then there's simply feeling bad without knowing how or why, and asking my loved ones to accept me without judgement while it blows through, as it usually does. How long? A week or ten days, a fortnight at most before things seem to readjust.

As for anxiety, there are shades and gradients there too, including:

Preoccupation: what I wake up with and carry into the day, past the toothbrush and the kettle; a concern that something needs to be done, but it'll be a tough task.

Worry: concerns and troubles that I'm at least aware of. I can name them, and I can tell myself either to reason them through, or knock the worrying on the head, which I'm able to do more or less successfully.

Rumination: when those worries grind on and downward, disappearing from the horizon of consciousness but accumulating force. The ruminating saps energy. I find myself possessed, needing to sit down, but I don't know what's really bugging me, I can't describe it.

(What I call) Anxiety: whatever's grinding away in the background stays there but it's grown and again, it becomes somatic, bodily, an experience beyond words. Sigmund Freud said that anxiety was fear without an object.

Fear: anxiety identified, given a name and an image. Otherwise, a natural response to objective threat, such as someone ridiculing me down the pub, an assault on my precarious dignity.

Paranoia: fear of a fugitive, multipolar threat. I've had this too, but even the awareness that it's paranoia doesn't relieve it. In extreme cases, the paranoia co-opts the awareness back into itself, recruiting it as further proof of "the truth".

Dread: outright terror, when I'm existentially afraid. *I'm dying! I'm back on that beach, drowning and alone!* Loneliness and meaninglessness at a cosmic scale. Thankfully this doesn't come often.

And by the way, these aren't as linear or hierarchical as the list suggests. Progression from one to the next is rarely logical or predictable. And it's not as if they're all illnesses either: some are perfectly human, natural responses too. Meanwhile I could also write a list of the random pops of happiness that arrive, the gentle unfolding of calmness, the spontaneous glow of wholeness or delight. But more often than not, trying to track and define shifts in my emotions is no more successful than trying to seal clouds in a casket or pin sunbeams to a wall. There's a constant flux between being ill and feeling well, a Brownian motion of circulating moods.

I add these as a way of repeating that asking for help begins with using the voice and finding words to describe feelings: it's a linguistic activity. And by the way, if you think these will help you put words to feelings if you're thinking of asking for help, feel free to use any of them. They don't belong to me, after all.

Perhaps it sounds a bit categorical or systematic to list feelings this way – an archetypally masculine way of rigidly ordering things (emotions) that are naturally ephemeral and often imprecise. But I should add that I'm not particularly conscious of "being a man" as I write this or, moreover, embodying what men are supposed to be – strong, purposeful, in control, certain and, in a very specific way, emotionally guarded. Armoured, let's say.

While we're gently probing some myths, I should also say that I'm not thinking about my six-pack (mine is more of a one-pack), or the dominant and successful position I hold in society: I'm a writer, a role that has never commanded much status compared with, say, athletes, rock stars or entrepreneurs. Nor do I view myself as irresistibly sexy and easily able to seduce women either – one of the ways in which male potency is measured. I've had girlfriends and loving relationships in the past but I found it quite hard to get a girlfriend when I was a teenager because I had an image of myself as weird and ugly: why would anyone fancy me? The splinters on this particular plank of shame have been rounded out as I've got older and understood more about myself and the mysteries of the opposite sex, our similarities as well as our differences.

Instead I track these emotional tremors and describe them knowing that they go beyond my own gender: they're felt and known by plenty of people I know, both men and women.

So when I look at this question of shame, it's through the eyes of a man, but I'm aware that we need to view it more widely – it's not as if depression and anxiety are uniquely masculine problems, after all. These days more women than men (6.8 per cent of women compared with

4.9 per cent of men) are diagnosed with generalized anxiety disorder in the UK today. Women between the ages of 16 and 24 are almost three times as likely (at 26 per cent) to experience a common mental health problem as their male contemporaries (9 per cent) and have higher rates of self-harm, bipolar disorder and post-traumatic stress disorder (see *Fundamental Facts About Mental Health 2016*.)[5]

Then there's what academics have defined as "the gender paradox of suicidal ideation", which shows that while men are more likely to carry the act out more violently, women tend to experience suicidal thoughts more frequently.[6]

Time to find out more about this matrix of shame, gender, illness and something else: crisis, which is one way of encapsulating what happened to me back in Berlin.

A couple of years ago I got to know someone who's as close to being an expert on all this as it's possible to be. Dr Luke Sullivan is a psychologist who works in NHS crisis intervention in south London, often dealing with actively suicidal people. He also runs a non-profit organization called Men's Minds Matter, which advances understanding of the overlaps of masculine psychology, suicide and well-being. Wanting to know more and put my own experiences in context, I called into his consulting room in Peckham one day not so long before writing this. One of the first things we talked about was the last entry on the list above: the problem of knowing that there's a problem in the first place.

Sullivan talks about how in his frontline work, he repeatedly sees people struggling with what he terms "the intolerable moment": facing a series of stressful events or situations in life – difficulties at work, an illness, relationship conflicts – which build up and can eventually become overwhelming. The result is a crisis in which suicide suddenly begins to offer some promise.

"I see this live in action," he says. "And it doesn't matter whether you have depression or not. If you find yourself in a position of emotional distress and it's persistent and intolerable, you will do anything to get out of it. It's unabating and it keeps going until people say, 'I cannot carry on if this is what it's gonna be like.' You can get that all of a sudden with multiple crises coming along all at once, or it can be a build-up, a persistent worsening of mood, a slow erosion that ends up in a space further down that line that people didn't see coming."

A certain blindness to their own interior world means that this all tends to be more dramatic and severe among men, Sullivan says.

"First of all you need to know you have a problem, and it's becoming more apparent to me that a lot of the men I see have no idea or conscious awareness that a problem exists. If I can't access my internal world and make sense of it, then I can't understand what it says, I can't put words to it and can't consciously put any structure around it... I just have something – something uncomfortable and unpleasant that could end up with me taking my life because I won't carry on like this."

It was interesting to hear from Luke that crisis – the result of a calamitous series of life events and stresses – is a greater causal factor in suicide than mental illness. He said that in the UK 72 per cent of all suicide occurs outside of mental health services, and many of those people don't have a mental illness.

"This isn't about mental illness," he added. "It's about life: a situation someone finds themselves in, where they're faced with a challenging, immediate, threatening situation that they don't have the capacity to manage, or are unable to find a resolution to."

That made me think about life – such as it was – in the sweltering August days leading up to my own breakdown. "Major depressive episode" was what got written down in my medical record, and it was a useful label for what I'd felt happening to me, albeit semiconsciously. Looking back, I can recall the intense surges of what I understood as anxiety, and what certainly felt like depression.

I also remember a related awareness that all I could do was soldier on with the objective struggles of my life as it was: a job I couldn't handle any more, the fact of a physical illness too (glandular fever), a relationship I was struggling to navigate and the immense heaviness of questions I was carrying. But the culmination was this rapid onset of suicide ideas, thoughts about methods and the overpowering obviousness of dying as solution to the intolerability of the moment I was living. A crisis.

Luke and I talked for an hour and a half, digging deep into these topics through his clinical insight and my lived experience. We also talked about how ways in which men are socialized can, given a certain set of circumstances, lead them to self-destruct. In a publication he recently co-authored, Sullivan wrote that there exists a dominant set of values and norms that define masculinity (or the behaviours of men) as we know them, variations on the theme of strength that include being "a fighter and a winner" and "provider and protector" and the retaining of "mastery and control". This model has elsewhere been called "traditional" or "hegemonic" masculinity.

These behaviours have roots that predate our own era: Luke also talked about the story of HMS *Birkenhead*, a Royal Navy frigate that in 1852 sank off the coast of South Africa, and was where the famous "women and children first" rule was first codified. Lacking sufficient lifeboats for everyone on board, the seamen gave their lives for others.

Since then the idea of strength in sacrifice has become one of the foremost masculine characteristics. However, according to Sullivan, it masks plenty of problems: the actual reality of men's lives amounts to "poor health outcomes, earlier death rates, illness and injury. There's something about the male gender that makes them very vulnerable. Suicide accounts for more deaths than homicide and road traffic accidents."

When he founded Men's Minds Matter in 2004, he was struck by the fact that nobody seemed to be paying attention to these issues. "It's like ignoring heart disease," he says.

That men are less fluent in and expressive about their own emotions than women is another popular preconception – but for Sullivan, it's something with grave consequences, because those dominant norms prohibit them from displaying or admitting to struggling.

"Insight into their psychological world, emotional experience and the capacity to function interpersonally to their optimum – these are the areas I see as most crucial when we talk about suicide. When you trace it back from adult life to childhood, there is less emotional development, awareness or literacy. So how do you introduce it as a language when it's not seen as an asset? There's the idea that emotions are weak, and that one should be stoic and emotionless. This narrative around emotion is totally bonkers," he says.

Bonkers is another word for madness, and one way of looking at madness might be the refusal to ask for help in order not to lose face, regardless of one's gender. "Help-seeking is antithetical to masculinity," he adds. "How do you show vulnerability when doing so may lead to you becoming more vulnerable?"

Being vulnerable versus "doing vulnerability"

It was interesting to hear Sullivan talk about vulnerability, and it might seem self-evident that the ability to speak openly about a painful subject is the first step in dealing with it: everything begins with asking for help.

But while vulnerability is a word we hear more and more since mental health and illness has become more a feature of popular conversation – a buzzword that captures an evolving attitude toward emotional candour – it makes me think not of men, but of women, and one woman in particular: Amy Winehouse. It's worth staying a moment with Amy to make sense of this "vulnerability" word so we can best make use of it, and avoid some pitfalls.

Maybe you too were shocked and saddened when she died suddenly in 2011. Personally I'd loved Amy Winehouse's voice and music, her tattoos, beehive and petulant virtuosity. Beyond her extravagant talent as a singer, what made her so luminous a performer was that she was so obviously in tune, literally as well as figuratively, with what she was singing about: what she seemed to feel in her heart was what came through in her voice, and the effect was almost mythically powerful. It all seemed so raw and sincere: performances from the edge of oblivion. It was a tragedy when she died a rock star's death at the age of 27.

Amy Winehouse was a performer who represented her emotional turbulence through music. It's important to remember that by the time we hear her singing, those performances have been mediated through recording studios, teams of managers and producers, through press releases, photo shoots, tabloid scandals and CDs with cool fonts and graphics, all designed to construct an image. In other words, what we as consumers get is a stylized performance of the torment she evidently felt, her rawness having been polished and commodified into something acceptable to the market.

But toward the end of her life there was a telling change. I remember reading reports that fans who'd seen her chaotic final concerts were disappointed and angry: they were upset that their favourite singer kept forgetting lyrics and stumbled around the stage, incoherent and intoxicated. The spectacle didn't correspond to the polished renditions of feeling in her recordings and videos. In fact, what the fans were seeing was a real, actual crisis unfolding live in public rather than the curated performance of one: a vulnerability that was manifest and actual.

The problem was that it was too real: too ugly, awkward and embarrassing to be palatable. By that stage Amy Winehouse was in the grip of severe problems: it's well known that she struggled with bulimia and substance abuse, and she was no more in control of her performance than she was of herself. It doesn't need repeating here that entertainment can be a cruel business, or that audiences expect value for money. But this story leaves us with an important distinction, which is the difference between being vulnerable (crisis) and doing vulnerability (performing). One is messy, unsightly and painful; the other is the kind of thing that plays well on Instagram.

So if we're to talk about genuine rather than performed vulnerability – if we're to be open to the fact that it exists, it's part of human life and that humans are prone to crisis, breakdown and dysfunction – then this distinction can be repeated, and it's something we can learn from the tragedy of Amy Winehouse's life.

Genuine vulnerability – in other words, when people really need help – is rarely pretty.

"Vulnerability" versus honesty

Nevertheless, it looks like this vulnerability word is here to stay in the contemporary mental health vernacular, and in any case, it's been around for a while. It entered the social conversation in 2010 when the US academic Brené Brown delivered a TED talk entitled "The Power of Vulnerability" (find it on YouTube) in which she discussed how we tend to hide shame and pain behind façades that end up imprisoning us. Brown's solution is opening up and letting ourselves be seen: "deeply seen, vulnerably seen", as she says, advocating vulnerability as a mode of living more fully and honestly. Her talk has since been watched tens of millions of times, suggesting that it touched a nerve, articulating a powerful and widely felt desire.

Since then vulnerability has been adopted into a vocabulary of personal growth and development that also includes "passion", the idea that we should all be enthusiastic to the point of erotic frenzy about something these days (saving the oceans by reducing plastic, say). There's also "authenticity", which relates to the belief that we're all supposed to be naturally and completely who we are. From a psychological point of view, this is a complex idea to say the least, but we'll look at it in a later chapter.

Alongside these, vulnerability appears to be a shorthand for emotional openness, an endearing new psychosocial equity, and it captures something of the contemporary warming toward mental health and illness. And no doubt it's good to confess to fears and despairs, or perhaps to having a diagnosis for depression or anxiety, taking meds, being unable to function, needing time out from work or struggling with social activities.

When, for example, the otherwise boisterous and self-assured grime MC Stormzy confessed to suffering depression, his testimony could easily be seen as an example of this hashtaggable #vulnerability in action rather than what it actually was: an admirable statement of humility or frailty. Superficially, this trend for vulnerability seems laudable. Yet one problem is that when there's social cachet attached to it, as Brené Brown's multimillion viewing figures suggest, it's easy to fake (this isn't, of course, to suggest that Stormzy was faking it; on the contrary). Even more problematically, the new fetish for vulnerability could also be just another way to feel anxious or even shamed for not being vulnerable enough: a commodified idea of openness. There's also the fact that vulnerability means more than one thing. It can mean being at risk of destitution: between 2009 and 2017, for example, the number of rough sleepers in the UK grew by 169 per cent, from 1,768 to 4,751, and I guess that these people would feel rather different about the way vulnerability is being fetishized today.

If it sounds like I'm being a pedant, I'd counter that we need to be careful with vulnerability because when it's misapplied or misunderstood it can easily end up obscuring what it's meant to reveal. We're back to Amy Winehouse and the difference between performing vulnerability and actually being vulnerable. The demand to perform her own vulnerability eclipsed her genuine need. She was trapped.

All of this is why these days I prefer a different word, one that needs less explaining: honesty. Asking for help because you're honest in your need for it, explaining how you honestly feel, communicating honestly with others – all of these swiftly cut through euphemism and sentiment. Being a language of directness, honesty acts like a disinfectant, revealing the gleam beneath the grime of pretence and self-deception, and banter, pleasantry and inference. It's less open to misinterpretation even if honesty is a blunt instrument that needs to be wielded cautiously.

For example, it's deeply honest to say to someone:

- "There's something I'm struggling with, can I ask your advice?"

- "I can't cope at the moment, and I don't know why."

- "Have you got time for a chat or a coffee, or a stroll? There's something I'd like to talk about."

- "I'm having a hard time at the moment. Can you help me think of some options please?"

Or most simply and honestly of all:

- "I need help."

These were the words I typed into a Facebook status update that day outside the office block, when in the desperation of crisis I was at the limit of my language and had no other syntax left in me; and even if later, when I was well enough to reflect on the moment, I was embarrassed at the alarm I'd caused.

Since then, I've tried to be as honest as I can be, with others and myself, alert to signals of self-deception or moments when I feel I risk manipulating others and corroding relationships by saying something unjust, or, just as important, not saying something important.

It's made life considerably simpler, for one thing. It also saved my life, this idea to ask for help that arrived in a critical moment. In a later chapter we'll meet a group of people who've made asking for help a cornerstone of their ethic, but for now, here's how they'd summarize everything I've said here: "Save your ass, not your face."

I sometimes wonder what would have happened if I'd done as much a bit earlier. Returning to the meaning and form of masculinity might reveal why I didn't.

The strength myth

In her 1990 book *The Beauty Myth*, feminist writer Naomi Wolf made the convincing argument that women's lives are subtly governed by the pressure to be beautiful, as if their entire worth rests on whether their appearance conforms to dominant aesthetic norms. Back then it would have meant one of the original supermodels: Linda Evangelista or Naomi Campbell, say; today it might be Gigi Hadid or Adwoa Aboah. When it's a currency administrated by men beauty becomes a tool to repress and control women, particularly when women have internalized the myth to the extent that they unconsciously conspire with it.

Three decades later, the same argument could be made about men's relationship to something we talked about above: strength, which is the marker of a man's potential in the sexual marketplace, his value at work, his status in the cognitive economy, but most hazardously of all, his relationship with himself. Living under the regime of what we might call "The Strength Myth", the man who feels himself to be weak – physically, intellectually or emotionally – automatically inherits a sense of shame. And often that shame is so unbearable that there's only one thing to do: hide it.

So far, so theoretical. What also tells the story is something that happened not so long ago when I was out on a winter walk with some friends over the South Downs in south east England. The morning had been bitterly cold, and some hours into the walk one of our group complained of having chilly hands; he'd forgotten to bring his gloves. I'd brought a second pair, so I offered them to him: "Here, have these," I said.

"Oh, thanks, but it's okay," my friend swiftly replied, shoving his hands in his pockets and trudging toward the horizon.

It struck me as odd, but I didn't ask why he refused the gloves. Even though for a few seconds I thought about turning his refusal, along with the expression of heroic suffering on his face, into a banter-y joke, I didn't want to embarrass him. Indeed, it reminded me of every time I'd said or done the same sort of thing, hiding what I needed or knew to be true within me, or how I genuinely felt, beneath a mask of composure, or a cool, studied indifference, and how doing so over the course of decades had led me to a position at the extremes of need.

Things you might need, but are afraid to ask for

- A hug

- Some advice on a decision you need to take

- Some money to tide you over

- Permission to admit you can't cope, or you feel anxious or depressed

- A break from the overwhelm of work

- Someone's attention

- To be listened to attentively for a while

- The ability to say something that's been on your mind: a burning desire, a guilty secret or a corrosive worry

- To spend time with people you've known for years, where you don't need to perform or explain anything

- A doctor to look at your health seriously and either reassure you or figure out what treatment you need

This isn't to say that my friend is a typically strong-and-silent, gruff or macho guy: on the contrary, he's kind, warm and thoughtful. But if it's a microcosm of the problem of shame and asking for and accepting help, then we can also look at the macrocosm – the way that men are supposed to be, or to say it more academically, the way masculinity is "constructed" in the West.

Working in the media, I've been part of that construction job. For most of my twenties I worked as a writer/editor on a range of music and fashion magazines: titles that are often concerned with "what's cool" at any particular moment in time. "Cool" is, of course, a value judgement, along with being a set of rules that, while being hard to identify, separates people into "cool" and "uncool". I spent a lot of my teens and twenties trying to be cool – going to cool parties, interviewing cool bands, wearing cool clothes, DJing at cool clubs. I probably even achieved the higher state of actually *being perceived as cool* several times.

In my thirties, meanwhile, I moved on from manufacturing opinions about bands and jeans and became a contributor to one of the leading men's magazines, and spent some time in this hypermasculine milieu. Along with celebrity interviews and fashion shoots offering fantastically aspirational lifestyles with sports cars, mid-century modern furniture, rare Swiss watches and so on, the stock-in-trade of this magazine was articles offering prescriptions, rules and commands on how to become a successful modern man: ways to get a six-pack or sculpted pecs or lats, tactics for picking up women, ideas on which sports cars to buy, strategies for corporate dominance, instructions on how to wear a suit or tie a dicky bow. Rules are handy for navigating life, but they can also induce anxiety.

It often felt like the subtext beneath these articles amounted to "Be like James Bond": drive a sports car, beat rivals, sleep with supermodels – or more simply, put money, power and sex before anything else. Implicit among these was the invocation to be strong, even if the strength in question was symbolic, or cosmetic – the appearance of strength. My guess is that most of the six-packs that end up on the front of men's magazines are rarely used for anything more purposeful than being photographed.

This magazine ran an annual awards show to hand out gongs to high-achieving men (athletes, rock stars, politicians, celebrities). I was grateful to get an invite to such a star-studded event, and every year I'd look forward to getting togged up in my suit and going along. I shook hands with Jay-Z, won a compliment for my suit from Brandon Flowers and to top it all, went for a pee in the urinal adjacent to Dave Grohl (I wondered briefly if his penis was larger than mine, and guessed that it was, if only symbolically. I didn't look).

The sheer density of success, glamour and blokey, banter-y testosterone in the building (the Royal Opera House) was so overpowering that, swamped in a champagne-infused shame, I'd usually leave the event and get a taxi back home to south London, drunk and sorrowful, compulsively reminding myself that "I'm not good enough." I didn't measure up. I was a failure, invalidated merely by comparison, or so I felt.

Back at my flat, in my mid thirties, freelance, single and renting, I felt very much unlike James Bond: doubting, at odds with these values, uncertain how to comport myself in this highly mannered yet subtly competitive environment. Asking for help in this kind of milieu is hardly the done thing: rather than saving my life it might instead have been tantamount to social suicide, and this is how "The Strength Myth" has functioned, in my life at least.

* * *

Nevertheless, for the past 20 years at least there's been an ongoing reappraisal of what it means to be a man, in the media and academia as well as down the pub. Recently the discourse has stepped up a gear with the emergence of terms such as "toxic masculinity", the revelations of ugly male behaviour uncovered by the #MeToo campaign, and the mounting critique of what's thought of as the patriarchy. Alongside these debates is a counter-narrative in search of new and broader ways to think about what being a man means, dismantling this burden of shame. The search is on for a model of being-a-man that is less laddish or brutal, more open, empathic and aware, more critical of traditional codes, along with greater fluidity in gender identities and sexual orientation.

It's about time, if only because it's too easy to look at the people who hold power in the world today – Donald Trump is the obvious contemporary example – and think that they alone represent what masculinity is: self-serving, narcissistic, misogynist and so on. However, most of the men I know – a number that easily runs to hundreds – are perfectly capable of acting like boisterous yobs at the beginning of a night out and like kind, broad-minded and empathic creatures at the other end of it.

As I've seen and known them, men are bewildered creatures too, and this supposedly solid edifice of stern masculinity is fragile, liable to fracturing under strain. The sensation of not knowing what to do or how to be that I had in sixth-form discos aged 17 returned to me at 42 when, holding down a stressful job, suffering glandular fever and wrestling with questions of life, love and identity, I was sliding toward rock bottom.

I didn't know what to do.

I didn't know how to be me any more.

I'm supposed to be strong and capable.

But I feel weak and lost.

Admitting it would make me look even more weak.

So I'll keep quiet and soldier on.

Until…

"Knowing what to do" is also an expression of strength which is, for better or worse, the cardinal quality of masculinity, the thing that, according to unspoken social and cultural codes, men are supposed to be. My best guess is that depression afflicts men in a particularly vicious way because it encrusts precisely that frailty, rusting away the chassis of strength and potency until it finally shatters.

What seems most critical among all of this is firstly the margin where masculinity's fragility meets the wound of mental illness: forces entwined in a yin/yang relationship that can lead men to suffer in silence and prevents them from asking for help, which itself can prove fatal. There has been a lot of attention paid in recent years to the problem of male suicide, but the most recent figures, from 2018, show a drop in the overall suicide rate among men, thankfully.

The second thing is that even though depression specifically seems to strike right on the nerve of what it means to be a man, it's a mistake to overemphasize mental illness as solely a masculine problem. Depression and anxiety are human illnesses, even if it's men who tend more than women to follow their thoughts and feelings more violently to the darkest of final destinations. And if we can wonder forever where these governing myths are built and maintained (the magazine stand in your local newsagent is a good place to start), what in turn governs both of these is something that takes us back to where we started: shame.

These days, I'm well aware that I'm neither James Bond nor an alpha male, a playboy, a bro, lad, metrosexual or any other convenient, explainable archetype of masculinity. I'm not even sure that "masculinity" exists other than as an abstract sociological concept, or if there are just millions and millions of "men" walking round with their own overlapping configurations of idiosyncrasy and identity. I'm one of them, but these days, when I need a hand with something, I know to ask.

* * *

It's taken me quite a while to write this chapter. It's been fretful, and to tell the truth I had to ask for help doing it: running my anxieties by a few friends; wondering if what I was saying was "right", or plausible, worth saying, or written stylishly enough. It's been tense, and there's a twinge in my shoulders. Truth is, I was afraid of putting pen to paper, or fingers to keyboard, and even as I reach this point where I'm moving to sum up my ideas on asking for help, why we don't do it and why we should, I'm still nervous about whether what I've written is good enough.

"Impostor syndrome" is one way of explaining this particular anxiety: the concern that you're insufficiently equipped or qualified for a particular task or role. It's a widespread, common experience, and I've known plenty of successful people who, in moments of gloomy introspection, have admitted that they've often felt like it was only a matter of time before someone – an unidentified authority figure, probably – tapped them on the shoulder and said, "Game's up, mate. Sling your hook."

If we analyze shame a bit further, we can see some other shadows in it: the tints of self-doubt or low self-esteem, the feeling that, contrary to what the shampoo ads say, you're not worth it. So, in a roundabout way, worrying about whether you should ask for help probably means it would be a good thing to do.

There may be many reasons not to ask for help, but in this field where shame overlaps with mental illness, and masculinity and femininity with vulnerability, and the requirement to be strong or beautiful can do more harm than good, something that's genuinely bonkers is the belief that appearing needy is worse than suffering in silence.

So if you're struggling: find the words that best describe the way you feel, use your voice and ask. Do it before you need to, then keep on asking.

Crisis, mental health problem, perfectionism – or all three?

Stacy Thomson is a mental health nurse and coach. She's worked both privately and for the NHS in frontline crisis and psychiatric liaison teams, dealing with people who've felt suicidal and sought help. Here she explains what to expect if you think you need help and you contact a crisis service or go to an Accident & Emergency department.

Over the last few years I have been in both crisis teams and assessment and psychiatric liaison teams, where I have worked with individuals who are in crisis. Part of the role includes the assessment of people who've been referred to NHS services via either their GP or another service provider. The role involves engaging with people in a way that helps them to confide about what is going on for them right now. Listening and asking questions is part of that assessment process. Some of the questions are designed not only to gauge what's going on for someone currently, but to help me get a sense of the person's background, including whether or not this has ever happened before. Getting an idea of the person's family, educational, career and relationship background really helps to build up a picture of the person and the potential difficulties they may be facing.

We need to talk about things that may be upsetting or difficult, including why they've come to be talking to me in the first place. People will often say "I can't cope any more, it's all too much and I don't know what else to do." In society today we are often overprotected from the harsh realities of life. Therefore, when something goes wrong, we struggle to find and apply the skills necessary in order to sit with disappointment and discomfort. This can leave the person feeling out of control, with most people developing an intolerance of uncertainty.

When that starts to happen, the central nervous system kicks in and a threat response is triggered, and all sorts of physical symptoms begin presenting: not sleeping, ruminating and so on.

It is important during the assessment that we ask questions around suicidality. This includes asking the person if they're thinking about harming themselves, and if so for how long and whether they've ever attempted

53

something in the past or if this is something new. But when we're looking at symptomatology, we can forget to look at the underlying issues that actually cause those thoughts and feelings in the first place: often entrenched belief structures that have been around for years, and which can be irrational, rigid and unhelpful.

Most people end up in crisis because something happens that escalates the situation and people reach out because they don't know what else to do, or they have reached a point where they feel they can no longer go on: "Help, I don't know how to deal with this." That is why I believe self-awareness is key: asking fundamental questions of what we actually think about ourselves, what we perceive about others and their judgements of us and how these things play out in our lives.

One thing that we always ask in an assessment is, "How are you sleeping?" In the later stages of really struggling, the brain is often thinking too much, or ruminating, and unable to switch off. Sleep is broken and the individual can feel exhausted. Physical functioning begins to deteriorate. We also may notice we are unable to focus or concentrate. The first thing that may be helpful is to help the person get some sleep, which is sometimes enough for them to feel better. This may include a short-term prescription of a sleeping aid.

What we often see is that people are unaware of their difficulties. They have very limited self-awareness and have let the depression or anxiety go on and on. They can let it spiral to a point where their self-esteem and self-confidence go down, and they start sabotaging themselves over and over again. They may get to a point where they think, "This is my only identity now," singularizing that one experience.

Fundamentally the first port of call is a GP. There are many self-help and psychology tools online but a lot of people just give up at that point, and it's also very hard to change things about yourself without help and guidance. The ideal scenario would be that we educate people from a very young age about the mind, and how we think, feel and behave, so we have an awareness and understanding as we grow up.

So many people who I come into contact with have, in my, view a behavioural or emotional dysregulation problem, but this often manifests into a mental health disorder. If we are able to identify the issues that affect how they're behaving and how they're feeling about it, we can then begin to work on developing healthier ways of coping and them accepting themselves.

On the other hand, a mental health disorder to me means something more severe, enduring and long-standing, which the person will have to work on for the rest of their lives, but which is recoverable. It takes a lot of effort to change thought processes and behaviours. The tendency now is for people to take medication, which most definitely can help individuals to recover. It will make them feel a little bit better, more themselves and more able to continue and move forward in their lives, but they may never get to the nitty-gritty of why they ended up in that situation in the first place.

I did my thesis on perfectionism. Paul Hewitt and Gordon Flett's Multidimensional Perfectionism Scale describes three dimensions: self-prescribed perfectionism (your expectation of yourself), other-orientated perfectionism (what you expect of others) and socially prescribed perfectionism (what you think is projected upon you, whether by society, environment, parents or peers). This one is the most commonly related to suicide. We naturally think that we have let ourselves down in some way and we're not meeting other people's expectations. We are also faced with social media that is providing us with a fake reality every minute of every day. The world is becoming more unhealthy. Consumerism is telling us we can have whatever we want, whenever we like it, however we like it. We walk around saying, "I demand you behave a certain way, I insist you go out with me and love me, I expect to get that job promotion." This is unrealistic.

If you can afford it, see a mental health coach, therapist or a counsellor. You might need someone who's a bit more forward-facing and proactive such as a coach, or you might need someone who just sits and listens, and who helps. Fundamentally there needs to be connectedness with another human being who says, "Look, I'll carry you."

One problem is that in the mental health space we're trying to find a one-size-fits-all scenario, but we're all individual, with different experiences, thoughts and feelings. That's why for me it's about understanding yourself: knowing how to catch yourself, recognizing things in other people and becoming more compassionate with yourself when things are starting to deteriorate. **www.impactcoaching.co.uk**

Who to ask?

– Your doctor

– Someone you trust

– Your best friend

– Your closest relative

– At work: your manager

– At school: your teacher

– Someone who you know has also struggled with a mental health
  problem

There may be a mental health clinic or crisis centre near you with people
you can talk to: do a web search to find one

Here are some other options:

UK
Samaritans
116 123 (24hrs)
www.samaritans.org
jo@samaritans.org

CALM
0800 58 58 58 (5pm–midnight)
www.thecalmzone.net/help/get-help/

The NHS also has a list of organizations to call if you're struggling:
www.nhs.uk/conditions/suicide/
If it's an emergency think about going to an A&E department.

Australia
www.lifeline.org.au
Call 13 11 14

USA
National Suicide Prevention Hotline
1–800–273–TALK
suicidepreventionlifeline.org

Germany
Freunde fürs Leben
www.frnd.de

International
www.befrienders.org

Next we'll look at somewhere else mental illness strikes – the body – and consider some ideas for mobilizing it in the service of recovery.

PS: Your story – did you make a start on writing yet? If not, don't worry. But here's a question that might oil the wheels: when did you start feeling this way? Maybe have a go at sketching out an answer.

CHAPTER 3

BODY PART I

A suggestion on what to do while you're waiting, beginning with a story

It was a Sunday evening when I realized I needed to begin again.

Sunday 2 November 2014, to be precise: the day my friend Greg and I drove 827 miles back from Berlin, crammed into his van alongside my bed and bike, some boxes, bags, keepsakes and all the other stuff I'd accumulated during my exile in the German capital. And when the realization came, I was standing in a cellar: a cold, cramped basement beneath a retirement home in the Shropshire town where I grew up. A place to stash my stuff, with a ceiling so low that even I, at 5ft 6in, couldn't stand up straight. I'd been at rock bottom a few months back – psychically as well as literally, on the Berlin tarmac – but it turned out I needed to go a few feet lower before the long climb back up could begin.

Lower still? Yes, it seemed that way. For years I'd dreaded having to return here because of penury or collapse, and now the day had arrived. Brought low in life as I was, it somehow seemed appropriate to be underground.

In the gloom I shoved the mattress into a corner, pushed the chest of drawers against it and slid a case of books underneath, economizing the space and sifting through the mystery of my possessions: a pestle and mortar (which I had no memory of ever using), two drills (who on earth needs *two* drills?); a pair of over-optimistically narrow jeans (unworn, of course); but also something that told a cheerier story: the brass medal they'd handed me as I staggered over the finish line of the Berlin Marathon, five years before.

All in all, stuff I didn't really need but couldn't let go of. I crouched down to survey the Jenga formation of boxes and bits and it looked pitiful, to tell the truth. All the more so when I remembered the episode of gleeful domesticity earlier that year when in a sequence of Ikea missions I'd splashed out on all this new furniture and begun sprucing up my flat, repainting walls, hanging pictures, feng-shui-ing the pad anew. Feeling, for once, "at home".

Warm memories evaporated in this chillier new version of reality. The lightbulb flickered and I banged my head on a rafter.

Stuff in storage, life on hold. November brings rain.

We locked the door, Greg drove me back to my mum and dad's, I went to bed and the next day woke up with questions:

– Well: what now?
What to do on this side of a breakdown, the sudden but necessary relocation and the abrupt breach with the friendships, places, the routines, patterns and coordinates I'd etched out in the last few years?
– What happens now?
I had no idea.
– *What on earth to do?!*

I stared at the walls for a while, then sluggishly got up: I'll go for a walk, I thought. Maybe an answer will come. I drank some coffee and chatted to my mum for a bit, then pulled on my coat and began walking the empty streets and lanes, all of them endlessly familiar and completely alien at the same time.

I did plenty of that over the following months as the winter thickened further, into the biting new year and on into early spring as the skies began to brighten and the temperature begrudged its way upward. Walking to the library, to the shops, to the fields nearby, along the railway line, up to the park and back again. Some mornings, bored of walking, I jogged round the garden 20 times, or pulled the saw out in the garage and began cutting the logs I'd collected from the nearby coppice. Yoga became intriguing to me, and I tried mimicking a few of the poses I saw on YouTube.

No answers came, but something else did: the vaguest of hints emerging from the simplest of routines. The hint came from my body and it said: move. Get up and get into your body. It's good for you if only because it proves you're not only a mind. Move the body, and the mind will begin to change.

And so, very gradually, it did. Walking lifted sombre moods a little, and sawing up logs gently rerouted the circuit of endless ruminating. "I need to make a habit of this,' I thought, so every day I resolved to do something physical: a few more logs, a longer or slower walk, even a few press-ups.

It was the first thing I learned on the other side of the crisis.

Do what's easy

There's naturally more to the relationship between mind and body, and what it means for dealing with mental illness, and in a later chapter we'll get physical again, looking more closely at the somatic dimension of recovery. But for now, movement, and making a habit of it, is the message. There are a few reasons for that.

In the first place it's easy to forget that you've got a body when depressed or anxious thoughts dominate your field of experience. And although I barely understood it at the time, this habit of walking, sawing and moving was proof of something I later discovered, and which is useful to know: serotonin, the hormone closely linked to mood, is often at its lowest first thing in the morning, but moving stimulates it. It's tempting to stay in bed, and often necessary. But on the move you're a body too, no longer solely a grid of thoughts.

But if this emphasis on the body sounds contradictory – after all, we're talking mental illness here – then something else I discovered is that one of the secrets to beginning to deal with depression and anxiety is to recognize how they manifest physically. There's some science involved in this, but the argument is simple enough.

In a pamphlet accompanying his recent book *Depressive Illness: The Curse of The Strong*, the consultant psychiatrist Dr Tim Cantopher made a persuasive case for seeing depression as a physical illness that arises in problems with the body's limbic system, one of whose functions is mood regulation. "Like any other physical system," Cantopher writes, "the limbic system has a limit and if it is stressed beyond this point it will break."

He argues that the type of person who tends to be afflicted with depression will, upon being stressed to breaking point, respond not by giving up or giving in, but by trying harder, pushing on and through.

"What gives way is the limbic system," he writes. "If you put 18 amps through a 13-amp fuse, there is only one possible result. Stress-related depressive illness is essentially a blown fuse."

Cantopher goes on to offer some sage advice about getting through depressive illness, emphasizing the importance of rest and then "avoiding any unnecessary challenges and only, where possible, doing what is easy."

"Once recovery starts, things get complicated," he adds. "You need to start doing a little more, but how much? The truth is I don't know. *But you do, because at every stage, your body will tell you* [italics mine]… at your body's physical limit at any point of recovery you will start to feel heavy and lethargic. For mental activity, you will find you don't take everything in. At social events you will start to find it difficult to talk sensibly."[7]

Mumbling incoherently, forgetting what someone just told you, feeling exhausted… all this may remind you of being at an especially tedious dinner party. Nevertheless, it is an accurate depiction of the mental and physical disorientation felt in the wake of a crisis, and it captures precisely how my life went in the weeks and months after asking for help, and for quite some time afterward. A year or more at least (and yes, recovery is a process best looked at in terms of years).

This habit of gentle walks and stretching my tendons into wonky yoga poses helped – if, that is, I could get upright in the morning, which sometimes took a Herculean effort. As months passed after my hit-the-deck moment back in Berlin, I wondered why this perpetual tiredness wouldn't shift. There were days when I didn't feel particularly fretful or glum at the level of describable emotions, yet I often felt as if I was wading through treacle.

At the same time, I had also felt an urge to get on with living life, leaving all this mess behind, and returning to my magazine-editing, late-night-carousing, distance-running former snazzy self. But, of course, it wasn't to be. As Cantopher so poignantly puts it, my body – the somatic me – was laying down the law on what was and was not possible. It rewarded me for movement but told me to slow down – and stay slow. The body has its own way of telling us what to do, and it usually has the final say.

This short chapter ends with a simple principle: once the voice is mobilized (finding the words to ask for help), then make your body the next thing to consider. The magic machine is always with you, after all, so collaborate with it to start building habits. Habits improve with practice, and practice – the things you do every day – is what will aim you toward a better state of functioning and, perhaps more powerfully than anything else, will describe the patterns of your life to come.

As for the here and now, maybe you're also finding that there's suddenly a lot of time to fill – if, for example, you're waiting for medication to take effect or you've sought help through public services (many of which have, sadly, been drastically cut in the last few years; the waiting times can be long). Certainly, in those answer-less, what-now? early days when I found myself once again living with my parents, I found the weight of empty time a heavy burden to bear. Walking lightened the load.

Lastly, if you're wondering what exactly to do with that body of yours, then check back with what Dr Tim Cantopher said above: do what's easy. If it's easy and you feel like it helps, keep doing it. Gentle walks, simple yoga stretches, some easy gardening. We'll look again at the value of building and maintaining positive daily habits in Chapter 10.

CHAPTER 4

MIND

Diagnoses, talking therapies and other ways of telling your story

Reflection

I try to do this every morning: stop for a few moments, sit and ponder; become aware of what I'm thinking about. Often on the edge of my bed, looking through the window onto the overgrown garden and the rooftops of south-east London beyond. Trace the outline of the horizon, watch as a magpie chases a crow away.

A fresh-air, clear-the-mind moment, and a useful habit before the momentum of the day begins to build.

And this morning I'm also wondering how to talk to you about the next subject, which is getting help, and looking at things like treatments, therapy and medication. This is a complex area since much of it is about the beginning of opening up between people – between someone who is suffering and someone, or others, who can help.

Maybe the question is about guessing where you might be in the movement toward recovery – near the beginning with the problem of knowing that there's a problem and wondering if you need help; or right in the panic and dread of crisis, just before or after this ask-for-help moment; or further down the line, on the path to getting better. Or indeed none of these.

So, I wonder.

What I know is that this morning is sunny. The last few days have been grey and damp, and the weather has begun shifting mood between summer and autumn. A reflective time. Photons lift my mood, and there's an unattached optimism in me. I mean, I'm not optimistic about anything in particular, I'm just optimistic. It's making me twitchy and perhaps that's why it's taken a while to collect myself and start writing and saying.

So: turn the phone off, close the browsers, set aside the to-do list. I need to start putting some of my thoughts down. Here are a few:

We often hear that mental illness should be considered no differently from physical illness. It's a cumbersome platitude these days, but it contains a useful truth. There's no shame in taking medications for the body, so there shouldn't be any shame in meds for the mind. They've certainly helped me, clearing the ground so I can start talking through problems.

Therapy comes from the Greek word *therapīa*, which means "healing" or "curing". My guess is that everyone would benefit from therapy, whether they're suffering or not.

If you can afford it, pay for it. If you can't, look for people who know something about these problems, who've maybe suffered themselves, and find out what services are publicly available. Many mental health services in the UK have been cut in the austerity regime imposed by the government, but people can self-refer through the NHS's Adult Improving Access to Psychological Therapies programme:

https://www.england.nhs.uk/mental-health/adults/iapt/

Therapy combined with medication is the standard method (or "modality") for treating anxiety and depression. In therapy, the talking itself is the cure. There may be lightbulb moments and flashes of sudden awareness where stuff makes instant sense, delivering relief from torment, but these are rare. Instead, the slow plod of talking and returning to troublesome topics is what effects the change.

The engine of therapy is a relationship between two people. The therapeutic alliance, as it's known. It might seem artificial when money's involved (a transaction: I give you money, you give me therapy), as if the relationship is contrived – but where else can you find a relationship that's as engaged and empathic? Therapy is something that oughtn't exist, yet needs to.

People can often have a lot of resistance to getting help. This is often to do with self-exposure (*what am I gonna find?*), guilt (*what right do I have to sit navel-gazing when others are starving or homeless?*) and shame or pride (*I don't need anyone else's help, I'll fix myself!*) Fair enough: these all make sense.

But therapy is best understood as a space to practise relating, new ways of feeling and thinking. The acid test is how it applies outside of the consulting room – back in the actual life you actually live.

I'm also thinking of another question that, with a worried expression on my face, I've asked a number of times. Am I going mad?

"As a rule of thumb, if you're worried that you're going mad, then you're probably not," said Dr Will Napier. "It shows you have insight."

Diagnosing the problem of diagnoses

It's safe to say Will Napier knows what he's talking about.

Will is a clinical psychologist who works at Esher Groves, a UK clinic specializing in the treatment of depression and anxiety. The clinic was founded by his colleague Dr Ian Drever, a consultant psychiatrist who I'd got to know after watching him deliver a powerful and convincing talk on the problem of smartphone addiction at a meetup run by the Minds@ Work Movement, the business and mental health network (I'm a member, and there's more about this organization in Chapter 9: Work & Purpose).

Between them Will and Ian have years of frontline experience in treating depression, anxiety and crisis, at the famous Priory hospital (Ian) and on the prestigious Harley Street (Will). But don't let that put you off: they know as well as I do that these problems never discriminate, and they're as much a part of our world as of that of the rich, famous and troubled.

I called down to see Ian and Will to find out what crisis looks like from the side of the consulting room where people in white coats sit (they don't actually wear white coats), but discovered quite a lot more, in particular that even beginning to think about asking for help is, for many, "a massive thing".

"The first contact I have with people often, after a referral has been made, would be an initial, no-charge phone conversation," Will said. "And the first thing I'll say is, 'Have you ever done this before?' It's a massive thing that you're even having this conversation – just getting to that point."

I wondered why people don't ask for help sooner.

"It's about recognition," Ian said. "People don't actually realize what's happening until quite late in the process: their sleep is disrupted or their appetite or memory goes, and they don't realize or recognize the warning that their body is flashing up to them, until quite late when there are so many lights flashing up in the dashboard that they just can't function. The body gives messages and it's important to recognize these and to respond accordingly at an early stage."

As I ran them through the chronology of my own crises and diagnoses, Will and Ian nodded silently. I got the impression that they'd heard many such stories.

"What strikes me is how incredibly typical this is and how the building up of events led you to where you were," Ian said. "It's almost always the picture that when someone was depressed or anxious, they were just carrying so much stuff on their plate. And often it arises quite insidiously over months or years where stuff just piles up – relationship, job, finance. This silting is very typical."

How full is your plate?

When I pause to anatomize it, this is the list of stuff that had, as Ian Drever said, "piled up" and led me to a point of crisis in 2014. It certainly looks like quite a lot when I write it down: a stressful job; a history of depression and anxiety; some perpetual, gnawing questions about the meaning of life and my identity; problems in my relationship; the absence of close family and old friends; a physical illness (glandular fever); an unhealthy relationship with alcohol.

One (or another) mistake I made at the time was believing that I could handle it all, push on through, master everything. It turned out to be another vanity.

Perhaps here it's worth doing your own audit of some common life stressors:

- **Work:** stress, long hours, insecurity, poor management, too much responsibility, under-or unemployment, being in the wrong job

- **Money worries:** paying the mortgage/rent and bills, putting food on the table

- **Problems in relationship and family**

- **Preoccupying questions:** the meaning of life, who I am, concerns over the future, the environment, politics and so on

- **Unhealthy lifestyle:** junk food, little or no exercise, poor sleep, too much alcohol and/or drugs

- **Over-healthy lifestyle:** too much exercise or time spent in the gym

- **Physical ill health:** a chronic or acute illness

- **Loneliness or an absence of sufficient "me-time"**

If you feel that you're struggling, remember: everything begins with asking for help.

I'd come with some specific questions to ask Will and Ian relating to diagnoses, treatment processes and the combination of medication and therapy – the stuff that usually follows after the "massive thing" of an honest admission of the need for help. Some useful overviews from these experts are included in this chapter. But what was more interesting was how our conversation looped around and between some of the received ideas relating to depression and anxiety, adding perspectives that can help separate sense from myths, for anyone for whom all this is a worrisome prospect.

There are, after all, some ideas worth mentioning: that medication is akin to the chemical cosh, sedating people out of their capacity to cause trouble, and that talking therapy can be ineffectual, infantilizing or even exploitative.

"In a narrow medical way, the medication and the talking is what treatment basically boils down to," Ian explained. "But for most people, the bulk of the treatment comes from the psychology – this seems to be true for two thirds of the patients I've seen. Medication would be a useful adjunct in some patients. Yet when people are severely ill is often when it is most difficult for them to do therapy because they are just so shut down. The irony is that you need them to get a little bit better before they can then make maximum use of that therapy."

Will used the analogy of assisted pull-ups to explain the relationship between medication and therapy: put simply, meds give people a hand up, and from then on they can begin to build their own muscle.

"The idea would be that if somebody could manage without medication, they would," said Will. "So a psychiatrist or GP would prescribe medication that would take somebody from being in a place where they can't even benefit from therapy, to being in a place where they can concentrate or relate enough to benefit. Gradually – ideally – you'd reduce the reliance on medication and increase the reliance on new behavioural patterns in their lives. You're not exactly curing something when you do talking therapy: you're coaching them in a new behavioural repertoire."

This raised the further question of whether recovery as we commonly understand the word (something with a finite endpoint) is possible, or even relevant, in this field. Answering this question is where, once again, conventional understanding begins to falter.

"We would always use the word 'recovery' guardedly," Ian told me. "Often it's about management and getting people well, but there's no cure. We can never guarantee, as in, 'get this episode sorted and then you're done, you'll never have depression again.' We would never say that."

Viewed from the extreme distress of rock bottom (where what's probably most important of all is the presence of caring humans, regardless of whether they are clinicians or not), this might sound dispiriting. But in another sense it can be liberating, especially in respect of the function of diagnoses and labels, how they can help or hinder us.

"Once you give someone a label and you say, well, there's only remission and there isn't a cure, then this is medical language for something that probably doesn't require it," says Will. "If you're seeing it from a structural point of view and somebody's suicidal depression is the result of everything going on around them and if you change those things, do you call it recovery, or do you just say things have changed so that they're now no longer suffering in the same way?

"Notwithstanding that there can be unlucky genes or a physical element. I don't think I've ever worked with anybody who has had problems with depression or anxiety that hasn't also had really substantial issues with their patterns of relating to people."

Making sense of medical words

What's flashing on the "Depression Dashboard"? Here are some definitions and explanations from Dr Ian Drever.

Depression is about a lot more than just mood. There's a whole constellation of different features, and mood is just one aspect of it. Mood is the headline act – but there are a lot of other warning lights that can suggest the depressive disorder is present, whether mild, moderate or severe.

In the ICD10 (International Classification of Disease) that we use there is mild, moderate or severe depression. In the DSM, which Americans use, there would be minor or major, with major corresponding to severe.

Symptoms include:

- Lack of enjoyment in life ("anhedonia": the inability to enjoy things)

- Disrupted sleep

- Disrupted appetite

- Diminished libido or sex drive

- Low energy

- A short fuse (perhaps you find yourself easily triggered and "kicking off")

- Poor memory

- Poor concentration: sometimes memory and cognitive functioning can be so poor in depression that people actually worry they're getting Alzheimer's because their memory just falls apart.*

*I'd add one more indicator to this: crying a lot, without knowing exactly why.

Depression and anxiety

Depression and anxiety are often like two sides of the same coin. If someone has some depression they almost always have some anxiety, and vice versa. Generally, one has the upper hand: a headline of more depression but with some anxiety, or a headline of anxiety but with some depression. It's very unusual only to have pure depression and no anxiety, or only to have pure anxiety and no depression. There's also mixed anxiety and depressive disorder, which is where the two are approximately 50/50.

Generalized anxiety disorder

GAD is classically characterized by what's called free-floating anxiety – anxiety that can hit at any time, as opposed to other types such as social anxiety, where it would only arise at social events, or agoraphobia, which occurs in crowded situations. Very few people have an illness that is perfectly textbook; there's almost always a spillover and some blurring at the edges.

Panic disorder

Panic is when anxiety is turned up to ten out of ten: a huge flood of anxiety, which is experienced both psychologically in someone's mind and also in their body. People will feel just utterly as if a catastrophe is unfolding. It can be so severe that they feel as if they're going to die, and often it's accompanied by a huge adrenaline rush: heart pounding, palpitations, trembling, sweating and even collapsing. It can look very, very alarming. People might think they're going to have a heart attack and die. Often an ambulance is called and they end up in hospital, thinking, "I'm having a heart attack," but actually it's "just" an anxiety episode.

Suicidal ideation and intention

"Ideation" is one of these psychiatric words that we never use in daily life, but suicidal ideation means having ideas and thoughts about suicide. Actually, most of us probably get that at some point in our lives, thinking, "Oh, is life worth it?". It becomes alarming when the thoughts become too active, with intentions and plans. That's when it becomes dangerous and when it would ring immediate alarm bells for psychiatrists or psychologists. Ideation turning into intention and then action can be very rapid or it may be a process that evolves over weeks and months.

We talked for an hour or so in the consulting room of Ian's clinic – it's the kind of space I know well from my own travels in therapy. There's a muted colour scheme, a box of tissues on the table, a few ornaments. More homely than the spare and brutally lit rooms one finds in hospitals or surgeries, it's a space for the mind to wander a little.

Meanwhile, when Will talks of the therapy process as "discovering ways to handle the dark forces, to handle them in a way that is more likely to be sustainable in the long term," it might sound like he and Ian are talking themselves out of a job; but in fact it tallies with arguments that have been going on for a while in psychology and medicine, such as the anti-psychiatry movement that began in the 1960s, or some of the views advanced by the psychoanalytical writer Adam Phillips. It's also echoed in something we've already talked about, which is the narrowness of the mental illness vocabulary: depression as a thing with many shades.

"There's a legitimate role for psychiatry and the medical paradigm on these things," Will says. "Certainly, in a fairly small number of conditions, there are things that you can identify – mental illness diagnoses that actually have reliable understandings. But I'm more interested in whether something's useful than whether it is, in some abstract sense, true."

Will is suggesting that, as words that map onto medical concepts or pathologies, "depression" and "anxiety" are useful, but they can also have the ultimate effect of de-autonomizing the person labelled – trapping them in a diagnosis they feel they can do nothing about.

"I spend a long time talking with people about what's actually going on in their lives, and you see that there's a reason why they're depressed. But in one sense there's no such thing as an overreaction: we react exactly in proportion to how we're perceiving. My clinical experience is that people think they're reacting out of proportion to a situation – being 'mad' or irrational – but once you actually get down to what is really at stake, you can understand where they're at. I work with people who are parasuicidal: considering whether they are going to kill themselves. Often one of the really difficult things about it is that they are suicidal because a pattern has built up in the whole of their life, starting with their family dynamics.

"We're having this conversation because we actually care about helping people in their suffering. But sometimes there can be unintended consequences to adopting mental illness language."

It turns out that there's an upside to this critical reappraisal of diagnoses, labels and concepts. Among the therapy techniques Ian and Will use is ACT (Acceptance and Commitment Therapy), a subset of Cognitive Behavioural Therapy, which enables people to distance or "diffuse" themselves from their troubling thoughts, as the popular practice of mindfulness does.

And then, in the process of change that medication and therapy can affect, it's even possible to reappraise sadness so that instead of seeming like a burden you think of it as nothing short of an "adaptive advantage", Will explains. "By the time we actually call something depression, it's a sort of runaway thing with a life of its own," he says. "But it's quite useful. The word 'emotion' contains *motion,* and emotion motivates motion: it gives you the oomph to do something you wouldn't otherwise do. So sadness gives you the oomph to withdraw, adjust and grieve, and get used to a situation. There's an adaptive advantage to doing that: if you didn't have the capacity to mourn, grieve, feel sad or get used to the fact that you just lost a particular status battle, you'd fight to the death. And that wouldn't be good for anybody."

* * *

What Ian and Will have said about the clunkiness of diagnostic language corresponds to my own experience of doing therapy, as do their views on how the things we call depression and anxiety are often about much more than malfunctions in the mind. Mental illness is a component of the storm that gathers into the crisis of overwhelm and suicidality, but it goes alongside many other things: the circumstances of one's life, one's bodily condition, responses to events at home or in the wider world. Then there's the question of finding meaning in life, and the complexity of that.

Perhaps it sounds easy for them to be objective and brainy about these things, while the subjective experience is a very private kind of purgatory: the lived experience, yours or mine, of being unendingly depressed or anxious. It needs to be repeated that these people do care in the sense that they're motivated by a desire to help, and their interest isn't only professional: they're humans too. However, this is where therapy comes into its own, with the work of making a personal and unique sense of everything: authoring a story that helps the sufferer give coherence to things, and authoring it in tandem with another human rather than in the garret of one's own mind.

What therapy does for me

I speak to my therapist once a week these days. He is an analyst in the Lacanian tradition, which means language is a central part of the process. When he explained his approach in our first session together, I rushed home and typed "What is Lacanian therapy?" into Google. The answers that came back might as well have been hieroglyphics, so I decided just to trust him and, seeing as I was handing over my hard-earned, to engage as fully as possible in it. Hiding in therapy is the first way of sabotaging yourself. It's also a waste of money.

But briefly: Jacques Lacan himself was a radical French psychoanalyst who built on the work of Sigmund Freud. The nub of Freud's work – the "psychodynamic" approach to therapy – was that we're ruled as much by the unconscious part of the mind as by the conscious, perhaps even more so, and that neurosis (mental illness) was rooted in this unconscious. One method of accessing this unconscious is through language, along with dreams, daydreams and slips of the tongue (calling your teacher "Mum" or "Dad" instead of "Sir" or Miss" is the classic "Freudian slip"). There's a big implication to the notion of the unconscious: that when the greater part of the mind is akin to the submerged part of an iceberg, we'll struggle to know ourselves completely and suddenly, we're not as in control of our destinies as we like to think (there's more on the different types of therapy in the next chapter).

As for my therapist, he speaks with a northern accent, he's a bloke and – in the manner of therapists being inscrutable "blank screens" to their clients – that is about as much as I know about him. If the blank-screen thing sometimes feels a bit weird, there is a function to it: it means the therapy is about me as a client and my conflicts and bothers. This is the way it works.

I've worked with him for over a decade now, and yes, it's often felt like work: when I haven't wanted to speak, or couldn't think of anything to say. Sessions starting that way are often extremely fertile after we've broken the silence, and I'm left wishing that we could carry on longer than the standard "analytic hour", which is actually 50 minutes. Sometimes "the work" begins with my mentioning some ripple in consciousness – a subtle sensation, some broken thoughts or a few frames from a dream sequence dimly remembered from the moment of waking. He listens, and he never tells me what to do: "directivity", as it's known, is frowned upon by the psychotherapeutic trade and one of the aims of therapy is to build autonomy in the client.

There are a few instances I remember well from the initial work we did. When I first showed up at his door in Clapham, south London, in around 2007 there was the guilt I felt about doing therapy in the first place: was I worth it, and would he be able to get his head around my emotional imbroglios and elaborate theories? I worried that I'd be too much for him – for anyone, in fact. We probably spent three months dealing with that question before setting it aside.

There was also, once I'd recognized it, a straightforward fear of telling someone *to their face* honestly how I felt, when I was slowly divested of a façade or persona. "Persona" is the word Carl Jung used for the masks we wear to negotiate life; these can be tools for survival, and my attempt to be a thrusting, A-type, man-about-town was one such persona. But as with the adage about celebrity, these masks can eat into the face, devouring and replacing an actual identity. My therapist gently and sensitively helped me to set some of those masks down.

This fear was, in fact, more of a terror – perhaps even a horror – of the emotional intimacy between me and this bloke sat patiently on the comfy chair opposite the couch. Sometimes it was frankly terrifying, all the more so because much of therapy is about this direct physical presence: the literal being-with someone and the meanings intuited from the field of somatic awareness – a stirring in the guts or flutterings in the heart. After all, it's the easiest thing in the world to be alone: rejecting the tangles of human relating, and limiting intrusions from the world by actually shutting it off altogether. This, as you probably know, is a guaranteed method of feeling lonely and unloved.

We've worked over Skype as well as in person, and Skype was handy during the years when I was living in Berlin and especially in the weeks running up to my crisis (though I had little idea that it was on the way). We've had stretches of not working together, working more regularly and at other times less so. A lot of what we've done has gone backward in time. Once we began looking further back into my infancy and teenage years as best I remember them, I was surprised at how much sorrow and hurt was permafrosted down there in hidden memory. Talking all this over revealed the stuff that hurts and the patterns I repeat.

Week to week and session to session we might, for instance, embark on a prosaic discussion of a dilemma, the analysis of a dream or some speculations on a session from last week, last year or last decade. Ten years in, I'm not "fixed", and if therapy has shown me one thing, it's that the prospect of being "fixed" isn't only a mirage, but also a dangerous idea. It also seems to me that therapy initially untethers people from fixed ideas, masks and patterns of thought and behaviour, and helps them find the comfort in uncertainty that Stacy talks about in Chapter 2: it helps them get on by getting unstuck. But that can be profoundly unsettling, in the initial work at least.

Over time the effect has been a change in me that I've felt as disturbing and reassuring simultaneously: this is what changing or being psychically in motion feels like. And if it sometimes feels like we are going round in circles – treading the same waters, returning to the same shames and furies over and over again – then I remember what he said to me once: "Therapy is like a coil. It seems like you're going round in circles. But you're moving forward."

A language above and beyond depression

I don't mean to give the impression that my therapist is God's gift to depressives, even though in many ways that's what he's been for me. A constant support for a long time now – through ups and downs, bumping along on the bottom and swerving though some big, real-life shifts: starting and leaving jobs, embarking on relationships and getting dumped, with realizations arriving and dreams evaporating, navigating the elusive "me" that shifts over time.

And while in those 50-minute slots I'm conscious of "doing therapy", I become less conscious of being depressed, or suffering anxiety. In part that's because he's shepherded me away from arid terminology into a vernacular of the human, substituting the word "despair" (because we all know what it means) for "depression", for instance. But it's also because in therapy those terms, again, begin to become radically unfixed, as do lots of others: ideas that we might hold to be categorically fixed such as "happiness", "strength", "shame", "man" and "desire". Norms get challenged, pulled apart and rebuilt with useful new meanings.

What I also mean is that what my therapist says may have some deep, Freudian psychological significance in it; but the effect can often be extremely direct.

"Some things get left behind," he said after I'd mournfully explained how an area of London I'd been affectionate toward – the rowdy bars and KFC branch of Clapham High Street – no longer held any appeal for me. After that I never went back to retrace steps or look for the ghosts of former fun.

"Writing is more for you than speaking," he said, after a long, mumbling digression where I explained in hesitant speech how I sometimes get y'know like sort of tongue-tied right? While hammering my deepest worries into a Word doc seemed way easier. My therapist rarely issues didactic pronouncements, but this one silenced me, which is what usually happens when someone tells me a truth I can't articulate on my own.

What he said about the superstition of breaking mirrors also had a powerful impact. One morning I'd shattered a hand mirror and was instantly convinced that this meant seven years of bad luck; another seven, in fact. "Well, it's interesting how some people think they can *limit* their bad luck to seven years," he immediately replied. My worries evaporated instantly. Life guarantees disappointment and trouble: accept it, because it gets easier when you do.

And, lastly, when we were drilling into some long-term anxiety for the nth time – an anxiety that had, at times, been so intense as to morph into paranoia, perhaps even psychosis; I had believed elaborate fantasies of conspiracy and threat – what he said imparted a huge sense of peace: "It's been entombed": locked away, un-returnable-to, beyond the claws of worry or rumination.

Conversations with my therapist show me the gap between what I think I'm thinking about and what I'm actually thinking about, and how I can better address them. We put words to things, and while there's the straightforward purging effect of bespeaking what's hidden, and the sense of being held when I'm in distress (there have been tears, panic and anger in our work), the baseline result of all this is an inner change, something I struggle to describe, probably because it's beyond words.

But in simple terms: I feel better, because I relate better. To him, myself and to others. We've generated a language for relating.

What therapy can't do

If it sounds like I am a fan of therapy, it's because I am. I've had a good experience of it, which isn't guaranteed, and I'm grateful for it. I've found it a critical exercise as well as an intersubjective one – something countercultural in the sense that while it may have begun as the search for a way out of despair, it's never since then been about a quest for happiness. Instead it critiques the "Cosmic Should" of happiness in the first place, admits that life is most real when it is at its toughest.

I haven't talked much about medication in this chapter, simply because it's something that really needs to be discussed between a person and their doctor (if it's on your mind, make an appointment with your GP today). Of course, I've heard people talking about their experiences, both positive and negative, of the different medications available, from SSRIs to tetra- and tricyclics and many more, and I've also heard the arguments against medicating; there are plenty of those too.

What I've personally found is that taking medications has removed a certain layer in the bandwidth of gloom, decluttering some cognitive space such that therapy can effect a change, and putting me at a distance from some of the more arduous depths of despair. In elementary terms, they've helped me function better.

What would I be like without them? Equally, will I (or you if you take them), be dependent on them forever? I can only address this honestly and say: I don't know. I'd rather not have to bother with brushing my teeth twice a day either but this, it seems to me, is one of the compromises I make in the gamble of living as well as I can. Plus, other people benefit from it too. I'd rather not inflict the dreadful state of my dental health on anyone else.

In the end perhaps all this raises another question: why didn't all this therapy and medication prevent the spiral into crisis and a major depressive episode – this crisis, burnout or breakdown? It's again something I don't have an answer for, other than to say that the suicidal impulse was, in one sense, a final breakdown in meaning that was necessary before I could begin to find new ideas to live by. It's been said that therapy is the only place in the world where we're relieved of the requirement to be happy or to enjoy (it was Jacques Lacan himself who said it): it's okay to be grumpy. It's also been said what is spoken between therapist and client – analyst and analysand – is better off staying between them. It rarely makes for good copy. Dreams may be fascinating to the dreamer and very useful in therapy, but it's tedious listening to other people's descriptions of them.

I'm saying that it'll soon be time to move on from talking about therapy and looking at why something is the way it is (reasons) and proceed toward what you can do about it (actions). Something else I've found is that it's not possible to make your way out of mental illness solely by thinking – you have to act too. Act, as in *do:* take action. That's what the next section of this book is about.

PS: your story: did you make any progress? If not, maybe put down some memories of a dream or a moment when things seemed to change for you. Sketch it out, as best you remember it.

PART II

RECOVERY

Addressing a range of topics and how they can be recruited into
dealing with mental illness and recovering from a crisis

CHAPTER 5

LEARNING & LISTENING

How learning accelerates recovery, and how I learned to learn again

Experience is the greatest teacher and the toughest lessons are often the best. So if you're struggling, it's a probably a sign that you're growing. How can you tell? By the fact that it hurts.

The pioneering American psychotherapist Carl Rogers once wrote that therapy relies on a person's "willingness to be a process": to get comfortable with uncertainty, not knowing all the answers, perhaps even letting go of the quest for answers (remember that *therapīa* is Greek for "healing"; it's a process rather than a destination). Maybe this also assists us in generating a definition of recovery: it's anything you learn to do that helps you feel or function better.

But first, learning and listening is what this chapter's about: the fact that we can learn, that there are books and people who can help, and the value of listening as a way to help yourself as well as others.

Walking

Today is a Saturday. It's early afternoon and I'm in a café in east London with Dawood Gustave, an extraordinary man who's been both a friend and mentor to me, often at the same time.

We met up a few hours ago in Islington and walked along the canal, then cut southward through the streets, stopping to observe the architecture or chew over some discussion point: Dawood usually turns up carrying a brainy-looking book or two. There's no endpoint for our walk – we're not walking to get anywhere specific. Instead we follow our feet and get lost in the moment, airing some thoughts and feelings. We could call it *flâneur*-ing, from the French word meaning to wander with no purpose, but that sounds a bit grand even if the spirit is identical. We're just hanging out, and since we're both restless people it makes sense to do so on the move.

Dawood is in his early fifties, he was born to an Irish mother and a Jamaican father and he grew up in the estates of south London. He left school at 16 and led a wayward youth but in his early thirties something unlikely happened: he won a place at Oxford University, eventually graduating with a degree in modern history. A career in law beckoned but rather than become part of "the establishment", as he puts it, Gustave took his learnings back to south London and worked for many years as a mentor at the Kids Company charity, helping young people navigate the grim everyday realities of inequality, social exclusion, racism, drugs and gang violence.

Dawood has been described as a leader, youth advocate and political figure, and even as Britain's answer to Barack Obama. He's charismatic enough to justify the comparison. These days he runs a consulting agency with some university friends, and he's a combination of conscious businessman, street mystic and social visionary, the product of two radically different learning systems: the elite, classical liberal education of Oxford and the Peckham campus of the School of Hard Knocks. Dawood has always seemed to me an example of the power of education in action, someone for whom learning has been the motor of social, intellectual and spiritual mobility. He's also seen me go through some dramatic shifts.

We first met in 2007 when I was pursuing my endeavours in triathlon, strenuously training and racing. At the time I'd also been writing a magazine feature on a wave of teenage murders in London, and Dawood arranged introductions to some young former gang members. When I called into Kids Company's Brixton HQ I was immediately struck by how positive a presence he was amid the good, the bad and the ugly of the young people's lives. One vignette sticks in my mind: about how the "youngers" would be shocked to see Dawood walking through the estates "one-up" (alone) carrying a book: the symbol of learning. The mere fact of his presence offered the possibility of a way out from the life of criminality and deprivation.

When we reconnected in early 2015, I was living with my mum and dad in Shropshire, scraping some emotional and psychological stability back together; ironically, at the age of 42 I once again felt like a grouchy and conflicted teenager. I'd visited London to see some friends and contacts, and Dawood offered me some work, inviting me to get involved in his new business. His presence and interest in me had a powerful effect: not only did I feel welcomed, but I even felt *liked*, which, it has to be said, can be quite something amid the hailstorm of compulsive self-criticism that seems inherent in depression.

"The Kevin I remember from 2007 was a triathlete, but also able to get outside the arrogance of being a triathlete and be present with these young black kids," Dawood says as we walk along Old Street. "Back then I remember you looking me in the eye and never seeing us as victims. But in 2015 I noticed that you were looking down: you were very boundaried, very poker-faced. I thought, this guy is obviously in pain, and I recognized that kind of pain."

Damaged seems accurate: it's true that back then, I was undergoing a drastic reappraisal of what I thought I knew and who I took myself to be, much of what I took for granted having been swept away back in Berlin, like pieces off a chessboard. I had a desperation for answers – how to live life, and how to deal with this depressed and anxious me – and as a result I'd become receptive to people who wanted to help. There turned out to be quite a few. So, I started listening to what they had to say. Just as importantly, I stopped arguing and complaining, and started doing it. Dawood had plenty to say.

I wonder what learning means for Dawood when it seems so central an element of his life: for as long as I've known him he's been learning or exemplifying, constantly engaged in the absorption or transfer of knowledge and ideas.

"It's like breathing; it means that I'm free," he says. "From other people's definitions of me, and mine of myself. If I'm not learning I'm not me. Not only literary learning but literal learning. I was growing up in survival mode, being bombarded by culture, music, food, difference, and learning became a necessity. Learning isn't just academic – it's the tool you need to survive."

"The thing is," Dawood goes on, "I like to mentor people, and I look for people who are going to help me grow too. I grew up in an age when men did that for other men, in a white working-class area; white working-class men would look after me. It's not about power or trying to control people, instead it's wanting to elevate them. And maybe I like people who've come though trauma. If you can get through that cycle and fight again, there's a lot of strength in that."

None of this is to say that Dawood has had what we'd term mental health problems; yet from the streets of Peckham to the spires of Oxford he's been through enough twists and turns to know that life is rarely plain sailing. He's candid about his history, knowing he could easily have ended up in a cycle of crime and punishment: "Sometime around the age of seven or eight I did a cost–benefit analysis," he says. "Do I become a badman, or do I go out and keep learning?"

He talks about how he was "hypervigilant", but years of study and introspection have enabled him to see the difference between what he calls "the guy I was, and the guy I used to act out." It built in him an acutely sensitive radar for human susceptibility.

Back in 2015 I was also struck by the evolving character of our friendship: it was empathic, where relationships between men are usually characterized as competitive and hierarchical, silently governed by codes of status, age and experience. On the whole men are resistant to taking advice from other men, let alone being looked after or out for by them, and it felt somewhat awkward to be taken under Dawood's wing for a while, like one of the traumatized "youngers" from Kids Company.

In other words, my pride took a knock. I was 42 after all: an adult, a man, and someone who's supposed to know what to do. But I swiftly realized a dose of humility was necessary.

In fact, it was a massive relief: a surrender to not-knowing. We're often told that being "empowered" is an intrinsically good thing, but sometimes it's wiser to submit and recognize what little actual power we have.

Somewhere near Brick Lane Dawood and I said goodbye to each other, knowing we'd be *flâneurs* again soon. We learned to learn from each other, and that's what makes these walks together so fulfilling.

Opening up, to others and oneself

It goes without saying that having a support network is important: a ring of souls to whom you can open up with your innermost despair, people who know you better than you know yourself, and can refer you back to a prior and perhaps more stable version of you when you're in the midst of a big shift. But let's repeat it nevertheless. I also discovered that regardless of one's age, it's also important to have mentors, guides and role models in life – people who've been before where you are now, and returned to tell the tale.

The experience with Dawood in 2015 turned out to be part of a pattern, and as the weeks and months passed, I kept meeting people, often randomly, who had something worthwhile to impart, something worth listening to. People who, when I told them what had been happening, said, "I know what it's like so here, do this. Try this. It'll help you, and here's my number if you want a chat."

One person counselled long, slow walks. Another, meditation. Someone else suggested living one day at a time. I wrote all of these things down and started doing them.

If I was receptive it was more by force of circumstance than decision. I had little choice other than to listen up and pay attention, to start looking and learning again. Equally, at the age of 41 I'd often had the feeling that I was somehow completed, had achieved a state of final formation as a person...

What vanity that turned out to be. Much of my existing operating system had been junked in the psychic upheaval I'd been through in Berlin. What I knew wasn't up to scratch and needed a dramatic upgrade.

So I listened, asked and then listened some more: to my friends, my therapist, people I met on buses and trains, in shops and cafes. I even listened to what my mum and dad thought about my situation. "Maturity," the psychologist Paul Watzlawick once wrote, "is the ability to do something even though your parents recommended it." Humility birthed an appetite for knowledge.

One evening, outside a recovery group whose weekly meetings I'd begun attending, another of these random, helpful people pressed a book into my hands.

"Read this," said Dave, a chain-smoking, caustically witty carpenter.

The book was *Why Am I Afraid To Tell You Who I Am?* by John Powell, who was a Jesuit psychotherapist. I read the whole thing that night, and its lesson can be learned from the title alone: why, indeed, when it's often the façades we construct and personae we adopt that (paradoxically) cause us to feel shameful, afraid and lonely. The book stresses the importance of relationships and the cathartic effect of opening up to others unguardedly and honestly, which, it has to be said, isn't easy or comfortable. It opens with the following lines: "How beautiful, grand and liberating this experience is, when people learn to help each other. It is impossible to overemphasize the immense need humans have to be listened to, to be taken seriously, to be understood."

Elsewhere the author writes about the mirage of the "true self" and with it the promise that if we eventually locate it, we'll be eternally happy. However, it goes on, "There is no fixed, true and real person inside of you or me, precisely because being a person necessarily implies becoming a person, being in process. If I am anything as a person it is what I

think

feel

judge

value

honour

esteem

love

hate

fear

desire

hope for

believe in

and

am committed to.*

(*It's worth spending a moment addressing each of these; perhaps doing so will add something to your story.)

I felt deeply consoled by reading this book from decades ago, sensing that I wasn't alone in my struggles. It was first published at the end of the 1960s and with its residues of open-hearted hippy optimism it has something of a utopian and idealistic tone. It could easily feel dated but it's all the more affecting given the often hysterical tenor of our own era.

Wise words, meaningful books and important lessons have a habit of arriving at auspicious moments, and maybe we only get what we need in moments of maximum necessity, when we're radically open. Other books such as this one, passed on with the guarantee of personal recommendation, touched me powerfully because I could locate myself in the tales they told.

They were especially useful compared to the blandly impersonal results delivered by web searches. Desperate for answers, I did plenty of googling but a certain lethargy came over me when studying blog posts with titles such as "How to Activate Extreme Self-Confidence and Destroy Chronic Anxiety and Fear", or listicles offering "Ten Ways To Overcome Depression Now!" They all seemed way too simplistic to be true.

On the contrary, since human needs don't change much, narratives on the conflicts inherent in being human, archetypal stories of collapse and redemption and the agonies of loss, fear, guilt and shame (all the really fun stuff) seemed more honest than the endless pages of "inspiring" Facebook memes, or glassy-eyed self-help manuals offering instant ways to get happy, fit, ripped, rich, lean or laid. Reading retrospectively in an effort to find some answers, I found my own recent story of confusion and breakdown was far from new, and not particularly original – and that in itself was reassuring.

* * *

I did a lot of reading and searching as spring slowly arrived in 2015, along with something else. One day, my friend Jon rang to offer me a room in his house in Bristol. Jon and I had been friends since we lived together at university some 20 years ago, and toward the end of March I hauled my Ikea bed out of the storage dungeon, instigated another round of brutal decluttering, rented a van and set off toward the M5. Here was a chance to rebuild some autonomy through the kindness of a friend, and also to give my tirelessly patient parents a break (from me).

Bristol: another new start.

Over the coming months, the pile of well-thumbed books began to grow. Here are a few more that helped, and which are worth passing on:

In *Man's Search For Meaning*, **Viktor E. Frankl** describes the possibility of finding meaning in life and a response to it under the worst possible conditions – the Nazi death camps, for example. Frankl survived internment in Auschwitz and this book formed the basis of what was later called existential psychotherapy. Its most famous quote is something you may have seen online: "Those who have a 'why' to live, can bear with almost any 'how'." This book revived my teenage affection for existentialism, but it is about the real-world application of these ideas instead of an exercise in abstract, salon-style pontificating. The basic lesson is: freedom causes anxiety because it means making choices against the backdrop of blank meaninglessness, and taking responsibility for what results. When there isn't any inherent meaning in life, then we're free to choose. Authenticity – another popular idea these days – means committing to those choices.

I chose to be a student for a while, committed to finding out what might help – after all, I needed it.

Then there was *Iron John* by **Robert Bly**. It was first published in 1990 and its strapline is "Men and Masculinity". This is a book I wish I'd read at the age of 22 instead of 42 because it prefigures the ongoing "what does it mean to be a man?" conversation, and subtly outlines the traps and pitfalls in the shift from boyhood to manhood: the same ones I'd unknowingly struggled with. More lucidly than anything else it articulates the problem of men and depression, and the links between masculinity, shame and grief, and using myth, poetry and psychology it paints a convincing picture of men as wounded and sensitive, aggressive and wilful simultaneously. It turns out my own generation of men weren't the first to wonder what being a man means, and *Iron John* offers a roadmap to this inner terrain.

So it turns out that humans have long wondered about the meaning of life and how to deal with the messiness of living, which is why a book by an even more ancient writer (about as ancient as they come, in fact) helped make sense of life in a time of vagueness and disorientation.

Marcus Aurelius was Emperor of Rome between 161 and 180, and his *Meditations* are a collection of thoughts on the craft and conundrums of living. You don't need to be a Roman to find something helpful in his writing; indeed, the scenarios he describes could easily be the kind of domestic aggro depicted in soaps like *EastEnders* or *Coronation Street*.

Taken together, these meditations are the centrepiece of Stoic philosophy, which advocates wise action, self-reflection and acceptance in the face of the inevitable – stuff that would easily benefit a common-or-garden neurotic such as me, and maybe you. The writings of Seneca and Epictetus, some 2,000 years before our time, also offer wise guidance in navigating doubt, fear and uncertainty.

Marcus Aurelius for depressed and anxious people

Here are a few Meditations suited to our enquiry:

To put anxiety over the future into relief: "Never let the future disturb you. You will meet it, if you have to, with the same weapons of reason which today arm you against the present."

For when the contents of your mind seem overwhelming: "Think of the totality of all Being, and what a mite of it is yours; think of all Time, and the brief fleeting instant of it that is allotted to yourself; think of Destiny, and how puny a part of it you are."

For when depression and anxiety have you trapped in an unending moment: "Time is a river, the resistless flow of all created things. One thing no sooner comes in sight than it is hurried past and another is borne along, only to be swept away."

When you feel like you're failing: "Do not be distressed, do not despond or give up in despair, if now and again practice falls short of precept." [8]

I went deep into the study of human fallibility: I read about Stoic philosophy, existentialism and positive psychology, and scrutinized baffling texts from Zen and Tao and some of the great narratives of religion. I began to understand more intuitively what Søren Kierkegaard meant with his investigations into "fear and trembling" and I devoured books by the groovy Oxbridge don Alan Watts, thinking that this bearded sixties dude was on to something with his meditating and transcendental visions in Californian ashrams.

In short, I understood something of the prehistory of human strife that stretches back from Frank Ocean to Joy Division to Black Sabbath all the way to the blues (music articulating the experience of depression before we called it depression) by way of Francis Bacon's depictions of humans in the abattoir of the absurd, then earlier to Hamlet and his suicidal contemplations, all the way back to Marcus Aurelius and the birth of tragedy, which was the first art form to suggest that life's a bitch and then you die (so try to enjoy it, if you can).

"Ah… all this is 'normal,'" I thought. "Being human hurts." Year after year, century after century, art, literature and music deliver up depictions and narratives of (what we call) depression and (what's known as) anxiety.

However, another effect of all this fevered scholarship was that I was spending way too long in the box room of my friend Jon's house, adrift in the expanding cosmos of my own mind. Then came another valuable piece of advice.

One day, urgently buttonholing Jon on some point of Kierkegaardian philosophy, he placed a hand on my shoulder, appraised me patiently and said, "Kev, look: this stuff is all very well in principle. But what counts is enacting it and being involved with the world out there." He pointed to the front door. "How about doing some volunteering, or attending a class, get involved in some groups? For one thing, mixing with other people will diminish all the distress in your own nut."

This too was advice worth listening to (and doing something about: I started doing some voluntary work) because it echoed exactly what I'd been reading in another book I'd like to share.

I've mentioned **Carl Rogers** a few times now, for a good reason. His book *On Becoming A Person* is a collection of his essays and lectures that explain his ideas on the dynamics of personal change. In the post-war years

Rogers founded the "person-centred" therapy approach, which emphasizes what he called the "self-actualizing" tendency in each of us. Put simply, Rogers reckoned that humans have a deep wish to grow toward the truest, most accurate and optimal version of themselves, and the function of the relationship with the therapist is to facilitate that. This is different to, say, the psychoanalysis developed by Sigmund Freud, which aims to illuminate the conflicts in the client's unconscious that cause them pain. In Carl Rogers's view, we get into trouble when we're not being our authentic selves. Even if that "true self" is, as John Powell suggested, something of a moving target, the important thing is the movement toward an ideal: the "becoming" part of "becoming a person".

To facilitate that movement Rogers suggests that the therapist can mobilize three key relational techniques:

- **Unconditional positive regard:** accepting the client completely and non-judgementally, regardless of whoever or whatever they are.

- **Congruence:** being mentally, emotionally and even physically "in tune" with the client such that they no longer need to deny, hide or repress what they feel themselves to be.

- **Empathic understanding:** one definition of empathy is "feeling into", and here it means the entering into what Rogers called the "private perceptual world" of the client. As far as possible feeling the things they feel and seeing the things they see, the better to understand them.

Naturally there's a lot more to Rogers's "humanistic" school of therapy, including the recognition that we all, somehow, need to feel loved and valued. And while *On Becoming A Person* is subtitled "A Therapist's View of Psychotherapy", you don't need to be a trainee shrink or even be in therapy yourself to benefit from reading it, because underneath all the theory it's essentially a book on how people change and grow – this process of "becoming".

And I noticed this happening to me as I wandered around Bristol, attending my tai chi class, picking up some work and interacting with others: I became aware of a break in the clouds; the perpetual, overcast feeling of doom began dissolving a little, bringing inklings of optimism, an emotional uplift, some inner modifications afoot.

Rogers's book put words to this experience: about clients undergoing therapy, he wrote that "They are not disturbed to find that they are not the same day to day, that they do not always hold the same feeling toward a given experience or person, that they are not always consistent. They are in flux and seem more content to continue in this flowing current. The striving for conclusions and end states seem to diminish."[9]

It may be terrifying to be in this kind of flux, never knowing how you'll feel from one moment to the next, emotions and thoughts pinballing around. But it often produces astonishing surprises, and that's why it can also be joyous. In the evenings I stared at the sunsets over Perrett Park, often overcome at the magnificence of the skies.

Listening

There's another important feature of Carl Rogers's work, which is to do with the relating and listening that my friend Jon talked about, and the essence of it is this: when you're emotionally distressed, you naturally need help, care and attention. But there's also a risk that too much of it serves to entrap you further in your own private sphere of turmoil and torment.

On the other hand, showing an interest in the lives of others (the simplest way of doing that is by listening to them) shifts the centre of attention away from the self and onto the objective world: the stuff happening beyond your skin. Doing so can be scary or bothersome, a bit like taking a cold shower (which is also good for depression), but it can also have the effect of temporarily reducing the internal cognitive chatter merely by dint of thinking about someone else.

As the Dalai Lama once said, "consciousness expands when we think of others". It can begin quite simply, by asking and then listening, never offering solutions, nor extending sympathy: just being with someone else for a while, where the "being with" is the important thing. There's little empathy without presence, after all.

Thinking about this stuff might make you realize how rarely we actually

– attentively, compassionately and selflessly – listen to others. At least, it did me. I recognized how I'd often cut in or interject – eager to have my say or express my opinions – not so much deaf to what the other person had to say, but blind to their need to be heard. So, I made it a habit to pipe down a bit more often, pausing before offering a reply. Try it out.

All this, I eventually realized, is what countless people had done for me while I was in the teeth of my crisis. So I began to put it in to practice, starting conversations at bus stops and supermarket checkouts, ringing friends up to ask how they were doing, practising the work of relating.

Anxieties subtly loosened their grip, a further layer of despair dissolved.

Included here are some ways to build a practice of listening:

Ways of listening

Listening to someone and taking an active interest in their concerns can help to create a meaningful connection between you and them, and can also help to take you out of yourself temporarily, diminishing the volume of your own inner monologue. Below is a basic primer on technique:

Levels of listening

1. Hearing
The attention continually scans the background hubbub but most of the aural information is disregarded. It wakes up when, for instance, someone calls out your name.

2. Listening-to
In dialogue where we're searching for an "in" into the conversation. For example, "Well I'm glad you mentioned that because *I* think...".

3. Listening-for
In dialogue where we're seeking confirmation of an existing view we already hold.

4. Active listening

A state of genuine receptivity: bringing the total attention, including mind and body, to bear on what the other person is saying and presenting. Clear the mind, be calm, breathe slowly (eight breaths per minute), allow the shoulders to drop and look the speaker in the eye. This is how therapists, counsellors and coaches are taught to listen, and what Carl Rogers would call "congruence".

5. Deep Listening according to Thich Nhat Hanh

"Deep listening simply means listening with compassion. Even if the other person is full of wrong perceptions, discrimination, blaming, judging, and criticizing, you are still capable of sitting quietly and listening, without interrupting, without reacting. Because you know that if you can listen like that, the other person will feel enormous relief. You remember that you are listening with only one purpose in mind: to give the other person a chance to express themselves, because up until now no one has taken the time to listen."[10]

Mindfulness and listening

Part of mindful practice is to notice sounds in the immediate aural atmosphere and your reactions to them, before returning the attention to the cycle of the breath. It's a useful way to sharpen your listening technique.

Find somewhere you can be alone, sit comfortably, close your eyes and monitor how the attention leaps to an ambient sound. Return it to the breath. Keep going for 5 or 10 minutes and if it works, extend your meditations to 15, 20 or 30 minutes.

Get into the group

The social conversation surrounding mental health and illness is coming into the open today, and more and more spaces are being offered for people to discuss problems such as depression and anxiety in the company of others. Andy's Man Club (www.andysmanclub.co.uk) offers meetups across the UK for men to get together to talk and share. Knowing that there's an especially intimate relationship between a man and his barber, Tom Chapman has led a campaign to help prevent suicide by offering grooming salons as places where men can open up with one another (www.thelionsbarbercollective.com). Meanwhile, the author Ruby Wax's Frazzled Cafés offer a similar network of spaces providing "a safe, anonymous and non-judgemental environment where people who are feeling frazzled can meet on a regular basis to talk and share their personal stories" (www.frazzledcafe.org). Sanctus, a start-up based in Shoreditch in east London (sanctus.io), also host mental health meetups, where three lead speakers share a story and the audience are invited to share back, then mingle and connect with others in a friendly and empathic environment.

All these organizations stress the importance of both speaking openly and listening to others. Here, Sanctus's community manager Rose Scanlon-Jones discusses how it works at the live events her company occasionally runs:

Sanctus's mission is to change the perception of mental health, and Sanctus Stories Live is an extension of that. How do you change the perception of mental health? By creating public spaces where people can openly and safely talk about their experiences of mental health and, crucially, hear other people's experiences. The aim is to remove some shame and mystery around talking about mental health.

The event itself is structured with three speakers and their experiences with mental health or mental illness: stress at work, a severe eating disorder or their journey through recovery, for example. Everyone in the audience participates in listening and gets a chance to reflect back to the speaker after they've shared. Then there's the opportunity for the audience to share themselves, just as the speakers did: standing up for a minute and, if they feel comfortable, sharing their own experiences of mental health.

The evening is hosted by me and our head coach, who is trained in holding the space, facilitates. It's safe and it's confidential as well, which is the most important thing. Honesty and trust are very, very important.

We give the audience a chance to get to know each other because as human beings we're already really, really scared to talk about mental health. We make the boundaries clear and address the elephant in the room. Who's feeling nervous? Who's excited? And why are we all here? We keep on addressing what everyone's feeling internally.

It's very easy to sometimes just open our mouths and talk, and sometimes you can get what we call a "shame hangover": "What did I just do?! That felt weird but I don't know if I'm safe." So the audience gets to tell the speaker that, "Yes, you are safe and I really appreciate your story and here's what I recognize in it, whether it's strength or resilience or honesty or passion."

For me it's important to talk to talk about mental health because it's the most crucial part of being a human. Personally I have definitely felt the short- and long-term effects of not talking about my mental health – not addressing it, not even acknowledging it. It enables me to eloquently express what's going on: feelings have words attached to them, but what does anxiety feel like? If I don't talk about them I'll never understand them and I'll just continue on this cycle of life.

What often prevents people from talking about their mental health is just not knowing where to begin and what's appropriate. We're bombarded with news of really tragic events going on all over the world, so no wonder people might think, "Actually, my problems aren't as bad as other people's. I should just pull myself up by my bootstraps and carry on." One reason why somebody might not talk about their mental health is because their peers around them don't, but if one person starts talking and then they bring a friend and then that person starts talking and their partner does, then there's a ripple effect.

Listening isn't a skill that society values much, and we need to learn to listen again. We get taught at school but we don't get taught to listen to people's feelings, to really hear them authentically, without any agenda or biases. To enter a space like Stories Live you have to accept the fact that your ego is taking a back seat – you're here to listen to other people and you've come to learn. It's a space to share, not a space to work. In therapy your ego can be massively there because it's a whole hour where you get to share everything that's going and the person in the chair will listen to you and work with that, whereas Stories Live is more a space for compassion and how we can as a group listen better.

Can you work on your mental health too much? Using the analogy of the gym and working your body too hard, then of course you can. I've felt that I have before: going to therapy, going to coaching, working in a company that talks about mental health, friends who talk about mental health... I also go to family therapy, I do journaling and I also have a whole community of a couple of thousand people DMing me every day asking me, "Oh I'm going through this, how can you help me?" I want to be a support for myself and others, yes, but is there a point where I have to draw the line? Of course, because otherwise I'd go bananas. The cure for me has been going into nature and leaving my phone behind.

Communities are massively important for mental health and mental illness because life is very individualistic now. Maybe you've got your Instagram, your side-hustle, you might be living in a big city and you're quite isolated, but in a community you're surrounded by people. Having five people that you can count on and know that if you picked up the phone and you were in a crisis they would help you – this is really important, a support system beyond a doctor, nurse or a therapist.

As for what's missing that creates the need for this, there are lots of little things rather than one big thing. With the breakdown of traditional family, friendship and work dynamics we're left with, "What now?" So whether it's a church, group of friends, book club, a spiritual place – somewhere you can grow where you can be around people who have similar values to you, respect your values and want only the best for you – is important.
sanctus.io

Back to school

There's a lot to learn from Carl Rogers and his person-centred humanistic approach to therapy, whether as someone who needs to be heard, as someone who wants to listen, or both. Some of the other thinkers I've mentioned – John Powell and Robert Bly especially – share this kindly and benevolent outlook, viewing we humans as bewildered creatures who are prone to doubt, despair and fragility, and in need of guidance and support (Carl Rogers initially wanted to train as a priest, though he later became an atheist).

It's wholesome, touchy-feely stuff, and as the spring of 2015 turned into summer I enjoyed bathing in the glow of "becoming", my fractured sense of self reintegrating as I listened and learned, did tai chi and made small talk with people at the Sainsbury's checkout. It reaffirmed my basic belief in the essential beauty of humankind. It also helped that I'd started taking a new med at the time – a mild antipsychotic that dampened down the more violent eruptions of anxiety.

The sun was shining. I felt more "chilled out." I even started liking myself a bit.

However, this isn't all of therapy, nor the only model for getting to grips with the problems of being that collect under the banners of anxiety and depression. And she might have meant it as a comic aside but when, a little while later, my tutor referred to psychodynamic therapy as "the dark side", she had a point. Eager to know even more about the magic interpersonal arts of relating, helping and being, I'd signed up to do a postgrad certificate in Humanistic and Psychodynamic Counselling at Goldsmiths College in London, where I'd graduated from two decades earlier. In case terms such as "psychodynamic", "psychoanalytic", "gestalt", "integrative" and so on leave you mystified, I'll explain what I learned about them here.

My tutor's point was that unlike Carl Rogers, Sigmund Freud didn't view human beings as misunderstood saints earnestly striving to actualize into wondrously complete selves, but instead as creatures ruled by the instinctual drives of aggression, lust, guilt and fear – the stuff that doesn't go down so well at dinner parties. All of this is hidden or repressed in the unconscious part of the mind, which, up until the early twentieth century, no one had properly noticed or got round to theorizing on.

The basic thrust of Freud's work can be summarized as "Where Id was, Ego shall be": the id is a wild inner animal and the job is to reconcile it to the ego, which is the self that we present to the external world with a freshly ironed shirt and polished shoes. The "I" that shows when I say "Hi, I'm Kevin," at the Sainsbury's checkout, for instance.

Freud codified the unconscious along with the practice of psycho-analysis, in which the analyst and analysand (client) journey into the depths of memory to locate the unconscious conflicts that result in "neurosis". Later analysts such as Anna Freud, Melanie Klein, John Bowlby and Wilfred Bion built on Freud's psychodynamic theories. Others critiqued it and still others flatly rejected it; but Freud's "dis-covery" of the unconscious remains a cornerstone of psychotherapy with far-reaching implications.

The image of a person lying on a chaise longue and chuntering about their mother to an out-of-sight therapist may be a cliché, but analysis as it's practised today remains a talking therapy that looks at early childhood experiences and the dynamics of projection (I feel angry at myself, but I project those feelings onto you), transference (what the client's relation-ship to the therapist reveals about their relationship to father or mother figures, for instance) and so on.

During the tutorials we also looked at the **existential therapy** approach conceptualized by the American therapist Irvin D. Yalom. On the face of it, signing up with an existential counsellor or therapist doesn't look much fun, since the therapy proceeds from what Yalom termed the "four givens" of existence, which comprise:

- "The inevitability of death" (yep)

- "The freedom to make our lives as we will" (so where to start?)

- "Our ultimate aloneness" (this one is easy to get your head round: simply use London transport during rush hour)

and

- "The absence of any obvious meaning in life" (wait... what?)

If that sounds enough to make anyone pathologically despondent, then the work of therapy is to help clients to confront and navigate these conditions, which are, after all, true. Since this therapy extends out of the prehistory of existentialist thought, perhaps it would suit someone with a philosophical cast of mind.

Next we studied the **gestalt** therapy approach, in which the word "phenomenological" features prominently. Don't let it put you off: it just means that the therapist and client work with the entire field of perceived awareness, from words that are spoken to intuitions and bodily sensations. These phenomena build into a useful "pattern", which is what the German word *Gestalt* means.

During the study of **transcultural therapy** our class saw some lively debates about the politics of race, gender, sexual orientation, faith, nationality and so on, and we got down to the question of personal identity, asking how (and even if) therapists and clients can come to understand each other across the divides of individual experience: for example, could I, as a straight white male therapist, enter into the experiential world of a POC feminist lesbian client – and vice versa?

This, of course, can only be a cursory glance at the dominant therapy approaches, and it doesn't include one of the most widely available techniques: **CBT (Cognitive Behavioural Therapy)**, which aims to effect change in a client by looking at the triangular dynamics between their thoughts, feelings and behaviours. Nor the relatively new **EMDR (Eye Movement Desensitization Reprocessing)** approach that is increasingly used to treat post-traumatic stress disorder.

And if you're wondering about "integrative", it means that a therapist or counsellor combines more than one of these approaches and others too (there are many more, including approaches that combine spirituality, faith, body and alternative ideas). Lastly, all of this can also be distinguished from coaching, a helping discipline that shares some overlaps with therapy but which is usually future-facing and more goal-oriented, premised on finding solutions and helping people get to where they want to go, in their career, for instance. Coaching is often based on models and frameworks such as GROW, an acronym that stands for Goals, Reality, Options, Will.

We fall apart alone and in private, but we heal together with others

This is what gradually dawned on me as I moved further on from the moment of crisis in Berlin, to my parents, and then to Bristol. Above all it is a learning process, and learning begins with listening.

So too it was confirmed during this course, which was an exercise in person-to-person relating as much as a dry study in theory. In our Thursday evening tutorials we'd study and then practise therapeutic techniques on one another, and the effect was a kind of "ambient therapy". I mean, I felt better simply by dint of doing the practical exercises, and enacting therapy with fellow students such as Anna, a committed existentialist with aspirations to becoming a bereavement counsellor, or Jon, a mild-mannered, studious chap who worked in an office by day and played in a death metal band by night.

And it seemed to me that regardless of the therapeutic model in question, it's above all the "therapeutic alliance" between counsellor and client that makes the change and effects the movement in someone struggling from worse to better, dysfunctional to enabled, fractured to integrated: human contact that shatters the glass box of isolation. Getting better is a social process as well as a personal one, resting as much upon the relationships we generate externally as the meanings we make internally.

There's another yarn I'd like to tell that will, I hope, illustrate this.

One Friday evening I caught a train from London Paddington back to Bristol. Travelling during rush hour from London is rarely a pleasant experience, but this evening was particularly fractious. I managed to squeeze onto the train and even find a seat and I noticed a thick atmosphere of unhappiness in the carriage. People looked tired, despairing and angry: quite reasonably, really. I thought about how many others on this train might in their own lives know the struggles I'd been having, whether they recognized them directly as depression or anxiety, or simply as being totally and utterly fed up with the daily grind.

Sitting next to me was a woman who I guessed was a little older than me, and we soon fell into an initially sheepish conversation, cryptically tiptoeing around what we both guessed was going on in each of us.

"Well, I've been... ill," I told her, euphemistically.

"Me too," she said. "Er, mind if I ask… What kind of ill?"

It took some gentle work to overcome a barrier of shame between us – it shouldn't be hard to talk about these things, even if it is – but once we had, the talk became extraordinarily candid and affirming. She told me she'd been in London visiting her support group, and recounted details of her own psychotic episodes and a suicide attempt. A little later, as she was getting off the train, she handed me a folded A4 pamphlet entitled simply "My Story", which was heartbreaking as well as being one of the bravest, most honest stories I'd ever read (and in 20 years of working as a writer/editor, I've read plenty).

We made friends and resolved to stay in touch. I also resolved to open my mouth a bit more often, start conversations, keep talking and keep listening.

* * *

At the end of this chapter I want to say: read as much as you can, start talking and keep learning and listening. When you find meaningful words and ideas that help, write them down and add them to your story. There's also a list of suggested reading at the end of this book.

CHAPTER 6

BODY PART II

From "I think, therefore I am" to "I move, therefore I become"

Time to get physical again – gently, still. In this chapter we'll look at ways of recruiting muscle, pulse and breath into the service of recovery, assisting the return from crisis. We'll build on the simple principle from Chapter 3 (where the body leads, the mind follows) but this time we'll also look at things the other way round, developing a mindful attitude toward the body and ways of keeping it vital.

No need for any extra anxiety, though: there won't be a revolutionary programme here, nor the promise of instant transformation. The golden rule is: do less than you can (don't strain), but do it more often than you'd like to. And if you're unfit, check with your doctor before doing something sporty.

For now let's start slowly and stay slow, with:

A moving meditation

Tuesday night: tai chi night.

I get on the train at New Cross Gate and travel north, arriving at Highbury & Islington for the 7 p.m. tai chi class I've been attending for a couple of years now. It's a beginners' group where we learn the four elements of this Chinese martial art. The class is run by Amaia from the Mei Quan Academy (www.taichinews.com), who, like all the best teachers, manages to be charming and stern simultaneously. It could easily be dispiriting when she's coming down hard on us because our stances are out of whack or we're moving too fast, but we know she's being tough for our benefit. Learning hurts.

In each class we work on qigong, a sort of moving meditation that stimulates energy through deep breathing, and the 24 Form, a long sequence of moves performed slowly; if you've seen people doing tai chi in a park, this is probably what they're doing. Then there's Pushing Hands (working with a partner) and Martial Applications, where we learn kicks and strikes, practising these elegant, cloud-like movements as if in combat. Tai chi originated as a fighting style and is basically slow-motion kung fu: that's the "martial" side. The art is in the endless process of learning and perfecting these movements, making them robust yet graceful, which is far more strenuous than it looks.

Each class we'll practise a particular movement over and again, connecting the position of the feet with the movement of the hands and the circularity of the breath. These movements have lyrical names such as "White Crane Spreads Its Wings", "Single Whip" and "Jade Lady Works The Shuttles" (I'm still getting my head round that last one). Learning each can be a frustrating experience, folding and contorting the body in a sort of physical origami.

In the beginning, lumbering through all this made me realize how poorly coordinated my mind and limbs are. Deeper into the practice, my agonized thinking-about-the-move has started to condense into a physical fluency – I mean, I don't need to think a movement through before performing it, and my body, more or less deftly, expresses it. In tai chi the body is never explosive or brittle as in, say, karate or ballet, and movements become more accurate the more softly they're performed. In some ways it's closer to swimming than anything else.

Then we chill. Every 15 minutes or so, Amaia instructs us to stop and set the body into a standing pose where we stay rooted to the ground, like those terracotta warriors. We meditate, breathing deeply from the diaphragm with the hands cupped over the lower belly to collect this obscure "qi", which means energy, or life force. Tai chi wasn't developed as what we'd call a mindful practice, but moment-to-moment awareness is one of the most striking effects it produces. I always notice that I've stopped thinking about whatever's been bugging me that day.

It's a social experience too: I'm in the middle of the age range in our class of 30-odd students, and there's plenty of friendly chat. We arrange ourselves into a grid pattern to practise the Form, peripherally aware of the others alongside whom we're moving.

It takes around seven minutes to complete the Form if we're doing so at the proper tempo. More often than not, we're done in a brisk four or five minutes, hopped up on the caffeine, email bother and techno-stress of the working day.

From her vantage point on the low stage of this school hall, Amaia scrutinizes us dispassionately, then issues the command to start over.

"Slower this time," she says. "Much, much slower."

At 9 p.m., walking back to the tube station, I notice I'm finally doing that: moving more slowly. I feel quieter and looser, stretched out yet somehow reinforced too. My feet are back on the ground where they belong, moving silently, one pace at a time.

So too are my thoughts calmer; I'm not ruminating too much. With these gentle movements, some of the cognitive strain has dissolved into my body, harmonized between mind and movement. I feel more like a total somatic system instead of a computer wobbling along on a separate mechanical chassis.

As for tomorrow, I'll get up and practise again in the park, before my thoughts once again soar off into the ionosphere of overthinking. I might also go for a run, which achieves the same thing. Nothing too fast or urgent, just 25 minutes around the streets, aiming into the wind.

There's one other failsafe way of overcoming the divide between mind and body as the sun comes up: get out of bed, roll up the blinds, fire up the tunes and just start dancing. Keep going for ten minutes, or the duration of three songs. Raise the heart rate and summon your inner James Brown or Beyoncé. Dance, as they say, like nobody's watching.

In any case nobody is, apart from that inner critic.

Strength & illness

As with walking and yoga, so too with tai chi, running, dancing: in their different ways these are conscious and nourishing methods of reconnecting the mind and the body, but of course they're hardly the only ones – almost any kind of movement will do that same thing. There are plenty of reasons to pay attention to the somatic dimension of recovery, foremost among which is that while depression and anxiety may generally be categorized as mental illnesses – maladies arising in the psyche – they almost always have a physical component. Certainly, depression as I've known it has sometimes felt like bodily as well as psychic pain – misery and dread deep in my tendons and organs.

Hence, it makes sense that the body itself can be mobilized into the recovery process, since it's partly the body that's malfunctioning. In fact, just as these days it's often heard that there's no physical health without mental health, there's probably no psychic recovery without physical therapy. But how and where to start?

That question came into sharp relief when one day in 2015 I got the bus into the centre of Bristol to buy some new running shoes, thinking that a new routine of pounding the streets would lift my functioning – physical exertion produces euphoric endorphin surges, after all. But inspecting the dummies bedecked in the latest technical apparel in the window of a sportswear retailer, I was suddenly struck by how absurd they looked: their bodies frozen into a dynamic ready-set-go position, at a 45-degree angle to the ground. Waxwork javelins exploding out of the blocks like Usain Bolt at the 2012 Olympics.

"No one actually exercises like this," I thought.

Indeed, looking back at the years in which I'd tenaciously pursued road cycling, triathlon and running, I began to wonder if the grimly intense, all-or-nothing, do-or-die approach to physical fitness was really the wisest path any more. Racing in the London Triathlon or putting in a respectable time (4 hours 23 seconds) at the Berlin Marathon had made me feel lean, strong and focused. But it wasn't exactly fun, and in the end it felt far more like work than leisure. It also made me feel lonely.

Still, it had begun well, and much of the low-key, generalized anguish and misery I'd felt in my mid thirties evaporated when I started training in earnest. I found that going for a run was the fastest way to shatter an anxious state, that swimming was a good match for a lugubrious mood and that cycling far, fast and high was an effective method of stretching the frame of my natural introversion. But being an elite contender in the sport of self-sabotage that I was, all this fitness and focus often turned into yet another reason to beat myself up: I'd feel panicked if through illness, injury or conflicting commitments I couldn't complete a certain run or ride in my training schedule. This was a pattern I saw reproduced in others. No level of fitness or achievement was ever quite enough.

So I gradually started to think it might be better to try something slower, gentler, with less of the huff-and-puff, the relentless pushing of myself in a bid to become the next Mark Cavendish.

This was what led me to tai chi. One day in the convenience store round the corner I saw a flyer advertising classes.

"This looks good," I thought. "I'll give it a go."

Enthused, I bought some baggy black trousers with dragon motifs embroidered down the legs (it's good to look the part) and innocently showed up that Wednesday night. Rather like going on a blind date, starting a new activity as a total novice can be nerve-wracking, and a frisson of anxiety accompanied me as I walked into the school hall in Knowle: had I overdone it with the trousers? Either way, the instructor was friendly and welcoming.

I spent the following week working on my basic tai chi standing pose, that I still practise now at my classes with Amaia. The following Wednesday it was a bit easier to walk into the class, say Hi and begin following instructions. I'd found something healthy and social to take part in.

In fact, those baggy black dragon pants helped: sometimes it's good to have all the gear and absolutely no idea.

Philosophy of body: finding an attitude and avoiding some traps

With all this I mean to say that while there's a straightforward and immediate mental benefit to moving your body, raising the heart rate a little and getting a mild sweat on, fitness culture looks intimidating these days, and sounds even more so. One of the unfortunate effects of the worldwide boom in personal fitness since the eighties (before which it was known simply as "sport" and "recreation") has been the transfer of the grand narrative of extreme athletic transformation from the gym into the cloisters of personal development, self-enhancement and LinkedIn-style career-building. In work as in leisure, nothing seems to be quite enough any more, and we're told we always need to be pushing beyond, achieving our "best selves", becoming somehow superhuman.

And with its emphasis on constant overcoming, resilience-building and striving to perform harder, faster, higher and longer, what an attractive narrative it is: *lift more iron or run faster*, it seems to be saying, *and you too can sprint away from the mundane, conflicted self you lug from home to work and back again, bro!*

There's no doubt that in some cases, the promise delivers. But if, when perusing Instagram selfies of buff dudes pulling their waistbands down to reveal sculpted abs or gorgeous gym babes parading iron glutes after a SoulCycle session, you feel these images are off-putting, even anxiety-inducing to the point of exhaustion – well, I'm with you.

Consider also marketing messages that have, at one time or another, been telegraphed by the world's leading sports brands:

- "Impossible Is Nothing" (Adidas)

- "Glory Through Suffering" (Rapha)

- "Power Your Performance" (Gymshark)

- "Just Do It" (Nike)

- "Never Stop Exploring" (The North Face)

And so on. Need a lie-down now? Just do it!

After a cursory glance at fitness culture these days it may feel that if we're not achieving goals on a par with Mo Farah or Paula Radcliffe, then we're abject failures – when in reality all we're looking for is a healthy way to keep active and stay in motion.

So here's a more plausible pitch, this time from Dr Tim Cantopher, who we met a couple of chapters ago: "The harder you push recovery, the slower it goes..." he writes. "As you recover, exercise will help you to feel better, but take it gently at first."

So how to be mindful when it comes to the body?

This has been a long-standing conversation between me and an old friend, Bruce Butler, who's something of a philosopher of the physical: he's a coach and sports therapist who today runs Motus Strength, a specialist CrossFit and callisthenics gym in west London. As schoolkids we did breakdancing outside the local cinema and went rock climbing together, in our twenties we DJed at rowdy parties and in our thirties we cycled the hairpins of the Alps and North Wales, our legs shaved and our Lycra scandalous. Standing well over 6ft tall, Bruce may resemble a mountain of muscle, but those pecs and lats hide a wise and critical mind. It makes sense that someone who for 20 years has been in deep and close relationship with the human body – coaching it to perform or rehabbing it back from injury – understands well the nuances of the soma, its individual quirks of strength and frailty.

I called into his "box", or gym, in Fulham to chat through these questions of transformation and embodiment, of narcissism, goals and the symbiosis of mind–body well-being. When it comes to the effect of exercise on mental health, he reckons there's no doubt that it works:

"The general systemic effect of exercise is as good as anything else for the healing or nurturing of your body," Bruce says. "But what I'm interested in is, what is normal? There's the happiness ideal: *you gotta be happy*. When prompted, most people these days will say they've had a depressive episode, but it may just be a normal variance, and they're not actually depressed. It's natural to be on that rollercoaster. I've had experiences like that, and I know it's probably just a normal fluctuation."

The atmosphere in Bruce's box is, like all gyms, intensely physical: we're here to move and train the body. But here it's an especially austere environment that, tellingly, has no mirrors, only steel frames with gymnastic rings (pull-ups are a big thing here), ranks of kettlebells, barbell plates, exercise bikes and racks of weight vests in case those pull-ups get a bit too easy. There are few distractions from the work, and the work, as Bruce sees it, centres on the whole human organism rather than the body in isolation.

"I'd say there's no division between body and mind," he goes on. "It's one organism. And regardless of a person's objective in coming to a gym, they will benefit from training. There are systemic health benefits, mental and physical. We don't know enough about specific cause and effect to say, 'Okay, this amount of training and nutrition will have a beneficial effect on mental states', but it generally will.

"You get better at what you do more of," he goes on. "It's really simple."

Motus Strength doesn't offer fat-loss or nutritional programmes, nor does Bruce weigh clients when they come in. Instead – and here's where we can learn something about exercise for its own sake – he encourages them to think about why they want to work out in the first place.

"Most of the population are influenced by the exercise industry in the media, where the big mistake is the use of exercise for specific objectives. Ask ten people why they need to exercise, and usually the reason will be weight loss or body-type transformation. But these won't lead to long-term health performance or mental benefits, because it's shackling exercise to an external reward or objective, which will eventually hinder your long-term health, or spoil your enjoyment of exercise.

"I've seen it many times: you've got your six-pack; you look great. So now your training can go. Where's the reason for you to train? It's disappeared. It's so shackled together, and your exercising is mainly a tool for appearance."

Narcissism – an excessive, compulsive concern with one's own appearance – is frowned upon at Motus Strength: hence the absence of mirrors. But in his mission to decouple exercise from external rewards (the approval of others, for instance), he's up against the power of the same black mirror we're all entranced by: smartphones and social media, Instagram in particular (there's more on this in a later chapter).

"Without a doubt, it's exacerbating the problem: people believe their own Instagram profile," Bruce says. "But it goes further in fitness, and the need for recognition is turning probably secure, stable people into neurotic freaks. That perpetuates their involvement with exercise in a negative way because it makes them train for vanity – for external reward. Everything is becoming ridiculous."

It certainly is, or has been for a while. But let's hang for a second, because the measures for generating a sensible attitude toward exercise, as Bruce sees them, are simple enough:

1. **Dismantle the idea of an external goal.** "Stop exercising with the purpose being your appearance, the reaction of someone on Instagram or to change your body, and train for some aspect of your own performance."

2. **Make it social.** CrossFit, which is a sort of competitive workout against others with measurable results, is one such way. "Put yourself in an environment where objectives are imposed upon you.

This is what CrossFit does really well. It builds community and introduces people to lots of new and different exercises. That will help people out long-term. The most powerful thing here is the fact that we've got a big group of people."

3. **Avoid exercise as an individuated, headphones-and-treadmill-plodding experience.** What this means in practice is: don't hire a personal trainer. "Personal training is one avenue of the individualized. But if you're in a supportive community and your needs are met and you're happy, then you won't be so insecure about having a tiny bit of body fat. If a personal trainer measures your body fat and says, 'Oh, you're 13 per cent – let's get you down to eight,' then you'll always be insecure about going above eight. Unfortunately, most of the fitness industry is equipping people with more neurosis. The industry norm is to get people ripped, cut, super lean, to have veins... it's not healthy."

4. **And lastly, do it for the sake of doing it.** In other words, the way kids do it: "Watch kids running around, jumping off boxes or playing football. They're not doing it to lose weight or improve their mental health, or anything else."

Finding a physical practice

In case you're still not convinced, here are a couple more mildly motivating body truths:

- **The fastest way to change your psychology is through your physiology.** So, moving can help change your mind, rapidly. This isn't my idea, by the way: I'm quoting Tony Robbins, the famous American coach. Some of what he says can come across as a bit Positive Mental Attitude-ish ("PMA" is a nice idea in principle but, for our purposes, exhausting in practice). But he's worth listening to.

And

- **Motion reduces tension.** If you're feeling anxious: get up, move,
  go for a stroll. This one comes from the legendary boxing trainer,
  Cus D'Amato.

Meanwhile, here's my definitive guide to undertaking different forms of
exercise in the service of recovery, in case you're feeling encouraged to
try something new and kinetic to requite your mind back to your body:

Running: start (very) gently and stay slow. Do it every day. If it makes
you feel better, keep doing it. If you don't like it, quit. Do it alone if
need be, and with others where possible.

Cycling and swimming: ditto.

**Triathlon, duathlon, Ironman, football, rugby, squash, all other ball,
racquet and team sports; boxing, kick-boxing, boxercise and
martial arts including but not limited to tai chi, karate, kung fu,
judo, MMA, ju-jitsu and aikido; HIIT, spin, CrossFit, bodyweight,
cardio, aerobics, acrobatics, acroyoga, Pilates and climbing;
5 Rhythms, capoeira, Zumba, Barre, ballet, flamenco, sober raving,
line, pole, Scottish country and all other forms of dancing; short-
or long-distance walking including walking round the park,
parascending, bog-snorkelling, cheese-rolling and ping-pong:** ditto.

I guess that you can see the pattern… While it's true that people may
experience a road-to-Damascus moment when they realize that, say,
round-the-world yachting or biathlon offers absorbing salvation from
whichever inner demons they're entangled with, no single sport, fitness
activity or leisure pursuit can guarantee it.

Nor is there a "correct" way of doing any one of them, at our level of
participation: we're all different, with varying aptitudes and configurations
of agility, toughness, bendiness, patience, rhythm and aggression. So find
what works for you, and develop a regular physical habit.

Then there's yoga, which is a bit different to all those activities above,
but the why and how is best explained by my friend Nadia, who I've often
talked with on what yoga can do for mental health.

Yoga: working on the acceptance muscle

Nadia Gilani is a writer who has been practising yoga for 20 years and is now a qualified yoga teacher. Here she explains what yoga has done for her and how it can help anyone.

It seems like yoga is everywhere these days. And although it was never billed as an aid to mental health, it can be and is, because what it offers better than almost anything else – re-embodying you, instilling an awareness of the breath and a distance from the perpetual tickertape of the thoughts – are timeless ways of getting or feeling better. Yoga was a mental health practice long before "mental health" was a thing.

People come to yoga for different reasons – improving flexibility, toning, losing weight, or because they've been advised to – but more often than not they end up staying for the same reason: the sensation of calm and the stronger sense of self that sets in with dedicated practice. I discovered yoga by accident when I was taken to a class as a moody teenager by my concerned mother, but it quickly became my thing, and since then it's given me an all-round sense of wellness, or served as a crash pad for landing onto in tough times.

Ironically, I didn't do it to improve my mental health, despite being unwell for many years (with eating disorders and later alcoholism) while practising it. The yoga was already in my life before things went wrong, and if at times I used it as a punishing obsessive-compulsive routine (perhaps a way of imposing control when I felt out of control), these days I have a healthier relationship with it.

Yoga can be a life-changing practice. It's no miracle cure (as nothing is), and nor is it easy. It's challenging physically, but also emotionally and mentally because it forces you to look at yourself, exactly where you are. And how many of us are comfortable doing that readily? The good news is – there's no rush, it's a life's work, so you can take your time and go deeper as and when appropriate for you.

Yoga will help take you inward, moving you away from what's in your head and tuning you into your breath. At its heart yoga is also a method for self-enquiry, which requires practice and discipline. In ancient India, where it originated, it was intended to be a spiritual practice, but my opinion is that spiritual experiences come to us when we're ready to receive them, so if that's off-putting and you just want to be able to touch your toes, calm down or de-stress, that's fine too.

With yoga you can explore stepping into your body. I instruct the people I'm teaching, rather than think what they might get out of a pose, to maybe consider what they might discover. Practise bending forward, backward, sideways, upward, downward, every ways, and that inexplicable "it" – whatever that is – might find you and keep you coming back. The shift starts to happen through breathing, moving and observing rather than forcing anything.

Yoga helps you cultivate and strengthen what I call the Acceptance Muscle. Even though I've practised for over 20 years, I've also been that person striving to get into a pose, panting once I got there, or flagellating myself for not making it. But over time I learned more about myself and realized the way I was approaching the practice was in fact the way I approached other things in my life: acting out impulsively, impatiently, lacking compassion. The more we practise acceptance of where we are, the more fluent we become at doing it and over time hopefully more inwardly still, more content.

This is why I believe in yoga for mental health because for people like us, the ones with way too much going on in our heads, it's possibly too painful to sit still. However, this is why meditation and lying down to relax both come right at the end of the class once we've exercised the physical body, which in turn can help still the mind.

To begin, try a drop-in at a studio or leisure centre and see what's on offer. It's important to find the style, teacher and environment that suit you. Some styles might feel like they ask more of you than others. The style I've been practising the longest is ashtanga (which is dynamic with lots of movement); I also practise yin yoga, which is a more still style, and I teach both. The real magic starts to happen when it pushes us to go inward and explore parts of ourselves we might not have previously been aware of. Making new self-discoveries, physical ones and others, can be humbling as well as exciting.

Everyone practises for different reasons: some like the physical level, others are seeking a deeper emotional connection (like me), and many want to take a spiritual journey. The bottom line is that we all practise because it makes us feel better, which is the only reason you need to get started.
Instagram: @theyogadissident

Body basics

Diet and wellness regimes come and go, and it's often hard to separate fact from fad amid the torrent of available and often conflicting information. But here are a few simple ideas for maintaining the magic machine that have made a difference for me.

Eating

In 2015, guessing my diet could do with an overhaul, I forked out for what I'd hitherto regarded as an appallingly bourgeois indulgence: a consultation with a nutritionist. It proved to be money well spent, and many of the suggestions offered by Jamie Richards, who specializes in nutritional health performance, really lifted my functioning.

"So: you're a carbohydrate machine," he said when I sketched out my general diet: cereal for breakfast, a sandwich for lunch, spaghetti for dinner, with crisps and biscuits in between. Carbs, carbs and more carbs, with a side of carbs. Richards reckoned that switching to a diet low in carbs and high in fats and proteins would help alleviate my often vertiginous mood swings.

There's some science in this process, and it's well understood these days. Briefly: eating processed carbohydrates such as bread, pasta and sugars causes a spike in blood glucose levels. Since the body doesn't like too much glucose, the pancreas responds by releasing insulin to damp it down. Insulin makes us drowsy, and drowsiness can bring dips in mood.

So we hacked my diet for a while, replacing all those bready, wheaty, sugary foods with eggs, fish, fats, oils and nuts. I started making spiced cabbage stir-fried in coconut oil, some baroque frittata variations, lunches of sardines and salad, and after coming to terms with the absence of carbs (it was exhausting at first but, notwithstanding a few manic relapses into Toblerone and Magnum Whites, I soon got used to it), I noticed a distinct improvement: a magical uplift in energy; and I felt both lighter and calmer. Those lunch-slump glooms began to evaporate.

"What we look for is foods that have very insignificant if not non-existent insulin-promoting properties," Richards says. "Salad and fish, good-quality poultry, limited amounts of good-quality red meat, vegetables, oils such as olive, avocado, all nut oils, plus herbs and spices, and eggs."

Meanwhile, some recent science has made a connection between depression and inflammation, which is one way the body's immune system responds to threat and stress. Richards reckons that the diet plan above can be beneficial for that too.

"Clean eating" (avoiding dairy products and processed food), the "Paleo diet" (ditto, along with no grains) and the ketogenic diet (rigorously avoiding all carbs) function along similar lines to the basic blood-sugar dynamic described above. These aren't for everyone – nor is any of this to demonize carbohydrates, which provide essential energy for the body.

There's one other key thing Jamie Richards recommends: avoid being a fussy eater, anxiously policing food intake and adding up every calorie. **jamierichards.co.uk**

Drinking

Or "staying hydrated", as it's known in the contemporary pseudoscientific argot. My instinct on this one is: trust your own instinct. Bodily and cognitive functioning decline when the body doesn't have enough fluid – everything gets slower, more torpid and achey – but remember, we're not trying to reach peak performance, just stable functioning. So follow your thirst rather than the guidelines printed on branded mineral water bottles; on the whole, people weren't dying of dehydration before the mass marketing of mineral water that began sometime in the eighties. The NHS suggests six to eight glasses of fluid per day and avoiding sugary drinks (for the insulin-related reasons above). If caffeine gives you the jitters or keeps you awake at night, cut down.

Sleeping

Sleep as long as you need (probably more than you currently get) and try to ensure that it's good-quality sleep. Install blackout blinds if you can afford them. Quit all devices and screens at least an hour before retiring, and leave them in another room. Then, a soporific herbal tea and maybe some slow, meditative breathing before lights out. Going to bed earlier than you might otherwise is helpful: as they say, "Hope is a poor supper but a good breakfast", and night-time or early-hours loneliness is the bleakest kind.

Vitamin B complex
Good for both energy and mood. I use Max B-ND from Premier Research Labs.

Get plenty of fresh air
Like your parents said.

Eat chocolate
Because it should be mandatory to indulge occasionally. I like Toblerone.

After movement, repose

Like lying down at the end of a yoga session, as Nadia describes; because passivity is important too. Learning to be still, and sitting with emptiness and even boredom, is the final element in this philosophy of body that we've developed, these workouts to bring the mind into the body and vice versa. What thoughts float through your mind when you practise that? Perhaps they'll provide something for your story, the feelings you intuit or the images that arrive (and while we're at it, that first-thing-in-the-morning dance routine: which three songs are on your playlist? Make a note of them too, add to them and programme the playlist to accord with your waking mood).

Finally, if all this sounds a bit random and unsystematic, let me add that in sickness and in health, being rigid with regimes has only ever served to create rather than assuage anxieties: these days I've got a better understanding of when I need to go faster or slower, or when my body needs more grunt (press-ups and running) or more float (tai chi and dancing). I try to listen to what it's telling me, interpret the messages accurately and act on them.

Sometimes the body needs to be wild too, injecting some disorder and sensation into the system: a mindless meditation. We can, after all, be too mindful – too much Zen, mineral water and awareness. The next chapter looks at what to do if the desire for wildness and disorder has become excessive, to the point of dependence and perhaps even addiction.

CHAPTER 7

SOBRIETY

What to do if and when self-medication becomes worse than the problem it's meant to treat. Plus a beginner's guide to Capital-R Recovery fellowships

The theatre of violent emotions

Friday, 12:58 p.m., in central London.

Through the entrance of the hospital facility, turn right and find the door.

Walk through and find a seat. Sit.

I'm in a room. Knuckles rapped on the table announce the start of the meeting, the mood grows quiet and everyone is attentive while others begin speaking, strictly one at a time. There must be 60 people here today – people in suits, people with tattoos, gay and straight people, people wearing clothes so fashionable it's as if they're from the future, people younger and older, silent and loud people, people who live in penthouses and others who live in shelters. All kinds of people.

Feelings start pouring out of the person talking. In hesitant speech with pauses and sobs the young woman is describing the waves of agony that have washed through her life of late, since she stopped drinking, which she had been doing heavily and daily for a long time. Now there are conflicts at home and problems in work but beneath everything is a tempest deep within, all the way through her skin to her organs and into her soul. Powerful feelings, but here they can be expressed and held, somehow diffused into the people present: no one's judging. After all, they've all felt that way too, done worse things and known the terrors of withdrawal and the emotional chaos, whether two months or two decades ago.

"It's f***ing hard," she says, struggling to stay lucid. A moment of gaunt silence.

She adds that today marks a milestone: her thirtieth day sober. She feels that it's a miracle. A cheer goes up, since it is. A tissue is offered and a hand alights on her shoulder and she adds a quiet thank you, then deflates back into her seat, emptied for the moment, flushed. Then it's someone else's turn to share and what we hear today – and might even speak up to share – are stories in the same naked tenor, confessions on shame fear rage guilt envy jealousy fragility lostness loneliness confusion heartbreak but also joy elation gratitude compassion love tenderness and you name it. The violence of all emotions, present in this theatre of catharsis.

The hour passes and the meeting winds to a close. People stand and hold hands in a circle, hard by the walls with the chairs shoved aside, and a prayer is said in unison: the famous Serenity Prayer.

The first word of the prayer is "God" (...*grant me the serenity to accept the things I cannot change*) but it's not necessarily addressed to the effigy of the crucifixion or to Allah, Yahweh or Jah, the white-bearded Big Guy upstairs, though some of the people might conceptualize their "higher power" that way. Individuals usually have their own notion: for some it might be Grandma. For others, a cherished dog. This power above and beyond might be love itself, and for others still this group of people is itself the source of strength in their battle with the bottle, or the rock, the wrap or the pin.

The meeting closes and everyone mills about for a bit, phone numbers are swapped and cups washed, then people move off and out, cleansed in some way: simplified and connected with one another and possibly something cosmic. An energy.

Hangovers

They won't help us on the path we're walking. For sure there's delight in the disorder of intoxication – the escape from time, the wild emotive visions and the instant empathy that makes you want to hug people (I'm pretty sure it's not just me). A pint or five is a guaranteed way to neutralize the distress of unvarnished everyday living, as is a toot, a puff or a pill. The downside is that tomorrow's reckoning always comes.

And no doubt you know the range a hangover can cover, from the mild Lambrusco giddiness that evaporates with the first cuppa to the grouchy thickness after a night on single malt. Further, and we're into blackout territory: the taxi you have no memory of getting out of and the scramble to fill in the blanks of what you did, said or lost: keys, phone, purse and maybe a job, a partner or something else you loved. If slaving through the queasiness, headaches and the shame is bad enough, then maybe the craving comes to reach for something to blot the pain out: more of the same; in which case the cycle repeats. Day after day on the hedonic treadmill.

I know this isn't easy stuff for us to talk about. People often get uncomfortable when questions of drink or drug intake are posed, and I'm one of those people. I'm also no warrior in the war on narcotics, nor a temperance fanatic: to everything its season. I've known to some degree the damage that drink and drugs can do, but in this chapter I won't guilt, horrify or lecture you into abstention. The message is that sobriety is a good match for mental health and for some people, sobriety is recovery.

These days I practise abstinence (and sometimes I even get it right) because in the past I've struggled, and there's been a dance between the me I've known as depressed and anxious, seeking respite and escape, and another me whose joyous hedonizing has bled into self-medication, even self-abuse. Sometimes a waltz, often a scuffle. Indeed, I can say, as I have many times before, that I'm Kevin And I'm An Alcoholic, that I've had to act on my drink problem. And when I've said it, I've also meant it sincerely, even if inwardly I've been uncomfortable with how fixed and certain that identity tag sounds: as with "depression" and "anxiety", it's been useful to help me navigate the terrain and learn some new ways to live, but it has only occasionally come close to providing a complete answer. Still: one day at a time, as they say.

So we'll talk mood disorders and intoxication here, or more accurately the value of its absence (sobriety), along with how misuse both leads to and often stems from (what we call) depression and (what's known as) anxiety. We'll also talk about some ways to deal with all this.

But we might also ask – what's behind the addictivity I've seen in myself and in others, and which you've probably seen in the world around: the compulsions that go beyond drink and drugs and into smartphones, shopping, sex and work? For those of us who aren't the connoisseurs who drink for taste rather than effect (apparently such people exist), why do we overindulge in sensation and psychoactives?

Well, because living raw is tough. Sigmund Freud said as much back in 1930 when, in *Civilisation and its Discontents*, he wrote how "by 'drowning our sorrows' we can escape at any time from the pressure of reality and find refuge in a world of our own that affords us better conditions for our sensibility".[11] This is exactly why intoxicants are dangerous and harmful, as Freud added.

Another confession before we get on with it: I first tried to get sober in 2013 when it became unavoidably obvious that I'd lost control of my thirst. The sobriety project was going pretty well until something else happened: the craft beer revolution. I'd long had an affection for ale in the upper ABV echelons, and especially for robust Trappist brews with transgressive names such as Lucifer, Judas, Delirium Tremens and Mort Subite ("sudden death"). So, with their enticingly cool graphics and kaleidoscopic flavours, those rinky-dink little tins, up to 10 per cent alcohol and beyond, craft beers proved too much of a temptation.

At least, that's one excuse I gave myself for the relapsing. But that in itself says a lot about how genuine sobriety works, according to the people who make it stick for years and decades. I mean that blame is what this chapter is also about – and it's also about how, when you stop blaming and start taking responsibility, things quickly improve.

You get better.

In fact everything gets better.

* * *

There are plenty of reasons to steer clear of drink and drugs, and some are prosaic (you save money and lose weight, drugs are illegal), while others simply amount to common sense: doing so clears away the sombre detritus of hangovers, mood swings and cravings. You feel lighter, clearer and more conscious, despite feeling a bit bored with all the empty new time that opens up. With alcohol there are plenty of ways of stopping, from programmes such as SMART Recovery (smartrecovery.org.uk) to community-based challenges such as One Year No Beer (oneyearnobeer. com), campaigns including Stoptober or Club Soda (joinclubsoda.co.uk), which is billed as a "mindful drinking" movement, and finally the application of white-knuckle willpower.

Today abstinence is on the rise among the young people whom advertising agencies categorize as "millennials", with almost a third of 16–24-year-olds practising abstinence.[12]

Many people are able simply and easily to stop, stay stopped and start again when they feel like it, drinking "normally". People like my dad, who I watch enjoying a modest bottle of stout while watching bass guitar tutorials on YouTube (Dad's in a band). However, many people with mood disorders or the complex overlaps of depression and dependence aren't able to, and as you might have gathered, I'm one of them.

But I wonder why, since my drinking history doesn't look so different from that of other people my age: nights down the pub from the age of 17 or so, clubs and bars in my twenties, dinner parties in my thirties and so on – perhaps because I'm British.

It's true that the UK is a boozy place in which to grow up, as our continental neighbours know. Sometime around 2011 while I was living in Berlin, my then girlfriend recounted a conversation with a friend in which she'd raised concerns about my enthusiasm for German beer. My girlfriend was Italian, and her attitude to alcohol was sensible: red wine goes well with meat, white with fish, beer with pizza. End of story.

"The reason he drinks so much is simple," her friend had said reassuringly. "He's British." Brits like to put it away, and my guess is that it's down to a certain shyness or emotional brittleness, an emotional inarticulacy that only loosens up on the far side of a few pints. Brits aren't very good at talking about their feelings. I can recognize it in myself, at least.

But while there are cultural factors, there are no biological or hereditary ones I can define, by which I mean no addiction as a behaviour learned from my family, none of whom have a problem with drink.

But the truth of drink's problem with me stands and, ordinarily, this might be the place to present a few of my own war stories: instances of blacking out, the things I've lost, people I've upset or disappointed, the times I've made a spectacle of myself. What tells the truth better is the less cinematic and altogether more dismal reality of where it tends to lead me: drinking at home, abjectly alone. There's an especially savage strain of loneliness that comes with being drunk and miserable on your own, totally void of love and connection. I can also recall glimpsing the madness in walking to the off-licence for the third time in an evening, long after midnight in fact, and suspecting that doing so might not be normal, certainly wasn't fun and definitely wasn't healthy. And lastly, while readying to square up to tomorrow's hangover, there was the feeling of being betrayed by this ingratiating substance that was meant to take loneliness away.

It's the same promise every substance makes, and while we're talking drugs, I'm grateful that I'm a total lightweight and never took many, aware enough that my psyche wasn't robust enough to handle them. I dabbled, as they say, while succeeding eras in popular culture rushed by, each with its associated intoxicant: speed with indie music, MDMA and cocaine with dance music, cannabis from drum and bass to grime. Running like the River Nile through the middle of all of this was alcohol.

Again – why? Or more precisely, why me? My best guess in the end is that drinking solved some of the radical aloneness and meaninglessness that I'd always felt deeply, a response to life that I'd never specifically written up as mental illness, but rather took as an existential fact: we're all alone, as Irvin D. Yalom says, and I'd felt painfully conscious of it. Drinking assisted me in breaching the membrane that divided me from others, and me from myself. It filled gaps and became a friend, which is why the betrayal hurt.

Over the years, amid periods of drinking and abstaining, of making solemn Sunday-morning vows to have a week off only for them to be broken by Wednesday, I've tried hard to separate cause and effect in all this: disentangling dependence from depression, figuring out the fuzzy logic of pathology and symptom. Did I drink so much because I was depressed, or was I depressed because I was an untreated alcoholic? And what does being an alcoholic mean, in any case – is it someone who sleeps on park benches, or someone furtively reaching for the second bottle of wine in an evening? I'd long searched for a root cause that, upon locating it, I hoped, would unlock everything, sort chicken from egg, and help make sense.

But no such luck – the search continues. But if this passage above says something to you about your own uneasy relationship between misery and pleasure, keep reading (feel free to skip if not). Plenty of others have been there before us, and figured out some clever responses to it. As I said, this chapter isn't about bashing the temperance Bible, but pointing out that there are things we can do to feel better in the chess match against depression and anxiety. Eradicating intoxicants is one such move.

The practical value of capital-R Recovery for people who find life hard

The story that starts this chapter describes the most recent recovery fellowship meeting I went to, last week. I include it because I've known how the young speaker felt.

Though these fellowships follow a tradition of personal anonymity, you've probably heard of them. They help people get clean and sober, and stay that way. They also do more, and the principles and programmes they follow could probably help anyone, whether addicted or depressed or whatever "normal" means these days. Functioning, let's say, if a little lonely.

Casting back to the first meeting I attended, I remember all too well the panic and shame I'd awoken with after yet another blank night out. Pale sunlight through the bedroom blinds illuminated misery and pain of an entirely new magnitude: I'd found a trapdoor in the basement of despair. I knew that something had to be done, finally, at last, because the problem had nagged at me for a long time. Years in fact.

I grabbed my laptop and searched the Internet. I found an address and, that freezing Sunday night in November 2013, pulled on a coat and chased for the U-Bahn, running the last few hundred metres up Hauptstrasse: it started at 7 p.m. and I didn't want to miss it. I walked in, found a seat, listened and sweated, understood little of what was said – this group seemed to be speaking in tongues – but around the room I saw a circle of serene, healthy-looking people who afterward came up to me and were kind, offering books and phone numbers as I told them what was going on and the way I felt: confused, isolated, terrorized by my own thirst.

An Icelandic guy said, "What's your name? Look, well done; you've taken the first step, it's gonna be okay." He gave me a book called *Living Sober*, a sort of sobriety guide for beginners, which was full of practical suggestions. I started reading it on the U-Bahn back home, and began doing what it said the next morning: staying away from the first drink and using the 24-hour plan (forget week- or month-long sobriety projects: do it one day at a time).

Over the coming weeks and months, it began to help. Stuff made sense. The dread lifted, replaced by a new and previously unknowable calm. I eschewed beer, and drank lemonade and also began reading what's known as *The Big Book*, which, since it was first published in 1939, has become the basic text for the recovery fellowships. While some of it sounded antiquated and other sections were baffling, with a heavy emphasis on God and strange-sounding spiritual matters, still others made a lot of sense, with their descriptions of the problems of alcoholic behaviour and suggestions on ways to deal with it. The sober living miracle began to happen.

Not that it was easy. Social events initially proved problematic: a natural fidget, I found myself unusually itchy and restless in company where everyone else was getting stuck into the sauce. But the feeling of being deprived didn't last long, and I started looking forward to going to bed with a clear head and waking up with one too.

Nor was it easy explaining to friends and relatives this recent change in conduct, not knowing precisely how to explain my sudden affection for lemonade and early nights. "I've quit," I said. To others I was more candid, telling them what I've told you above. While most were supportive, I noticed how this new and rather more boring version of myself made some uncomfortable. I guessed that to some extent we all feel guilty about drinking, with hangovers as the price for the pursuit of pleasure.

But above all, what I discovered was that seen as a presence – a choice, something to cultivate and maintain – rather than absence or denial, sobriety could be almost magically beautiful. I felt cheerier and more energetic, and over time the effect proved to be cumulative. Once the boozy fug dissipates, the vision clears and the inner emotional turmoil calms down, and with it came a much clearer understanding of what my conscience was telling me.

One cliché that often circulates in the fellowship rooms is that the good thing about getting sober is that you get your feelings back; and the bad thing about getting sober is that you get your feelings back. In other words, sobriety cuts both ways: not all feelings are pleasant but acknowledging them in the clearest of lights is to address them for what they genuinely are: real feelings rather than synthetic ones, alchemized from a bottle or a pill. You may feel angry because you are actually angry; but you may feel delighted because you're actually delighted, too. While I can't say I've been completely sober since that panicked dash in 2013, I've nevertheless found that having long stretches of sobriety has been positive for my emotional health, if only because it has allowed me to assess my inner state as it is, in all its actual rawness. Plus, while I'm hardly immune from saying dumb things to people while sober, I'm likely to say more of them when drunk. Sobriety helps to strip out a further unnecessary layer of shame.

In the rooms they told me to keep working the Living Sober techniques, stay aware and, most importantly, "keep coming back". So I did.

* * *

Of course, you don't need to drink or do drugs to experience dread – the outright terror of being conscious and in pain – but the people in rooms such as I describe above have a word for it: that "gift of despair" we heard about a few chapters earlier. A gift because it impels you to do something, make some changes. Which changes and how, exactly?

To explain I've enlisted another friend, Jo: an ex-Berliner who's been clean and sober for almost a decade now. Jo and I have sat in the rooms together, taken tea and gone for walks. She's seen me go backward and forward on this track of recovery, and talking with her can help put my experience into the context of her own. On this occasion I called round to her flat in west London, where the kettle was on. It was time for some "spiritual sunbathing".

"What keeps me clean more than anything is connection," Jo says. "With my higher power, and speaking to my sponsor as often as I'm able to or I need to. I try to engage with the fellowship as much as I can, carrying the message elsewhere and going to meetings as well. A big part of that is random acts of kindness that nobody knows about. I think of it as spiritual sunbathing."

We'll explain what some of this terminology means, but in the first place let's address some of the signs suggesting that a pleasure has become something more worrying, which include drinking when you don't want to drink, or when you've lost the power of choice over a drink or a drug; when you can't stop or when one drink is never enough, or when an internal nag ("this isn't healthy") has become too insistent to ignore. However it's defined, the ultimate effect is, according to the fellowships, to bring someone to what they call "the jumping-off point": can't drink (because it will be too painful) and can't not drink (likewise).

"For me, the way to know that you've got a problem is when you stop showing up for life," Jo says. "When you don't care about things that used to matter: you've started disappointing people and yourself, maybe you've stopped eating and your every waking thought is about finding something [a drink or a drug] outside of yourself to escape yourself. That's the time to raise your hand and say, 'Actually, help me because I don't know what to do any more.'"

What prevents people from doing that?

"Pride is probably the biggest thing that prevented me from doing it for years. But when the pain of staying the same outweighs the pain of changing, you know you need to make the change. The trigger is different for everyone, but recognizing that something has to change is what it is at its very essence."

I've often asked Jo what being an alcoholic or addict really means. After all, I've used the terms myself because it's the protocol in these fellowships for people to refer to themselves that way ("My name is _____ and I'm an _____"), even if these days there's other vocab that says the same thing: being *a person with alcoholism* or *a problem drinker*, for instance. Bear in mind that DSM-5, the standard American directory of psychiatric illnesses, no longer lists "alcoholism" as an illness but "Alcohol Abuse Disorder" instead.

"Self-identifying is important for me because it was the first time in my life when I actually owned it, and I was responsible for myself," Jo explains. "Okay, I've done this, this is who I am: an addict. Ever since I was a child it was obvious that there were traumas and the way I responded was by acting out, whether with food, people, places, things or, later, drugs. It stemmed from trauma, but taking responsibility for it and saying, 'Right. It stops here, with me,' is where recovery started. It helps me to understand.

"Owning it is a way for me to find ways in which I can not act out, and not hurt myself. Because that's at the very core of my addiction:

self-medicating and ultimately self-harm. It's also about saying, 'Can you help me to understand myself, so that I can live a better life?'"

The help Jo mentions in these fellowships involves precisely that: meeting and being with others, listening to them share and sharing along. "It's about being of service to each other. One of the biggest revelations to me was hearing people talk and identifying with them. I thought I was so different from everyone else, but for the first time in my life, to walk into a room and hear people say, 'I actually know how you feel' – that was how I knew I was home."

It also means working with a programme of successive steps, usually with a mentor figure (known as a sponsor), which first involves admitting that the problem exists, then self-enquiry, considering the facets of your character that lead you to excess – a tendency to anger, for instance – and what you can do about them. They also involve prayer and meditation and, later on, letting others know that they too can ask for help if they're struggling.

The ninth of these steps involves the process of amending: going back to the people you hurt while you were drunk or wasted, and saying sorry. Setting aside blame and taking responsibility for your part in whatever went wrong: blinking first, as it were.

I must admit that when I was going through the steps with my sponsor a few years ago, this prospect sounded unappealing to say the least. I'd felt sorely wronged by life – a victim of circumstance and biology, of the cruel world, the demands and selfishness of others.

"So, let me get this straight," I said to my sponsor, somewhat outraged. "Go and say sorry to *them*?"

It didn't really compute, and definitely didn't seem fair.

"Yes," my sponsor said. "Go sweep your side of the street."

He fixed me with a kindly expression and the discussion ended.

I bristled for a while, raging inwardly, but eventually girded my loins and began: with family first, then friends I'd upset, colleagues for whom I'd caused problems… and the list went on. I said I was sorry, and I meant it, and in doing so, another modest miracle occurred: it no longer mattered who'd been "right" or "wrong". I felt my conscience clearing, and understood the blame and resentment I'd held for the toxic agents they are – energies that enchained me to the hurts of the past – and glimpsed the truth contained in a paradox: that taking responsibility brings freedom.

The more you take, the freer you get. This is what Jo means by "owning it".

Along with cultivating daily habits (prayer, meditation, journaling) this is also what "working a programme" means, and I've seen the extraordinary turnarounds it has effected in countless numbers of lives.

Yet if it all sounds like an intriguing but inessential byproduct of trying to stop getting pissed so often, well, I understand, but again: apologies, because there's a bit more to explain. The God thing: spiritual matters, questions of faith. Uneasy stuff. Let's stick with it.

Anonymity politics

I often look at Jo with admiration. Her recovery from addiction has been resolute, studiously crafted and, the way she tells it, absolutely necessary. She got it first time, which doesn't always happen when people wind up in these rooms. If at times it's stopped working for me, it's because I stopped doing the daily work: when I've tuned out, got bored, over-thought things, or simply drifted off. I've often turned to Jo for advice too, along with a few of the other self-declared recovering alcoholics and addicts I've become friends with.

These people often have something in common: a certain serenity in their comportment. They avoid over-involving themselves with people, places and things, instead sticking to what they know is theirs to look after. "Step into a hula hoop," one of them once said to me. "Everything inside is what you can control. Anything outside, you can't control. So let go."

And I've noticed something similar gradually infusing my own life. For one thing, merely attending meetings and listening attentively somehow reduced my sense of self. The effect is astringent. I mean that the incessant wants, needs and fears of my ego, and the attachments it makes, the terrified inner me with its restless search for gratification, seemed to get whittled back to a more modest measure, and I'm momentarily released from their grip.

All of which is a colossal relief, especially in an era of excessive concern over the politics of identity. The great leveller in these rooms is the recognition that regardless of age, gender, status, orientation, wealth, talent or influence, we're each of us in the end just alcoholics or addicts (or both) trying to stay free from intoxication.

"There's something really powerful when you're all sitting together and you're all equal," Jo says. "When there's no hierarchy. We're the most seemingly dysfunctional people in society, but when we get together in these meetings, there is a certain level of respect all of a sudden we just give to each other.

"The ego falls away: I love that freedom. Again, the process of working the steps helped me to become less me-centred and more God-centred. This whole world isn't about us. The fellowship has helped me to be selfless, putting others first. I haven't got the answers. I tried that route. It didn't work."

Similarly, these people don't blanch when spiritual matters are talked of. Does God exist? I have no idea. But what seems true is that God, faith, belief and especially religion haven't really been palatable to polite society for decades as the soul of Western man and woman has drifted toward the promises of individualism and self-gratification, notions of empowerment, satisfaction and achievement.

Faith and spiritual practice seem to help when those promises prove empty (beer never gets more tasty the more it is drunk; usually the opposite), or where the individual meets its limits. Setting oneself in relationship with a universal something brings perspective.

"If there's anything that I've learned in recovery it's that everyone needs to believe in something, whatever that looks like," says Jo. "I used to always feel alone, especially in my deepest, darkest days after using. Now, I don't feel that any more. I hated myself and from the age of 14 to 27, I had suicidal ideation every day. That's just not my reality any more. I've turned around because I've put the work in. It's not a bed of roses every day, but I also have tools now to deal with it."

But in the end, the most powerful value of a fellowship is in shelving shame for a moment and opening up with others, as they do the same. Sharing thoughts and stories, and recognizing that we're all more alike than we are different.

"I picked up drugs because I needed something to fill myself. But in recovery the beauty is in doing the unpicking, the finding who you are. Everyone's recovery journey is different, and recovery for me is whatever gets you to feel better about yourself and to make your situation better. Working an honest programme, you say, 'I need help,' and ultimately, the fellowship will help you to ask for help."

Talking trauma

The price of entry is, of course, renouncing a pleasure, though by the time most people get to the point of asking for help the substance in question has long since ceased being pleasurable. The fellowships are based on the belief that addiction to drink or drugs, or sex, gambling, work or food (along with cross-addiction, where a person substitutes one substance for another) is an incurable and progressive illness, meaning it gets worse over time, and can end in death. It's true that there aren't many elderly drug addicts around.

There's another view, of course. In the past I've discussed this subject with Dr Jane McNeill, who specializes in trauma therapy using the relatively new EMDR approach (Eye Movement Desensitization and Reprocessing) and has worked in the treatment of addiction. She says that addiction can be looked at through the disease model, which assumes that once something has developed into a problem it is very difficult to unlearn the coping behaviours: using drugs or alcohol to manage distress. But it can also be seen as a learned behaviour, which implies that, like most learning, it can be un-learned.

Either way, Jane says, "It seems that once people have developed the addiction and have gone beyond drug or alcohol misuse and into abuse and they are pharmacologically addicted to the drug for a long time, most people find it very difficult to go back to moderate use. It's hard to unpick those behaviours."

"If you have an immediate relative who has a substance abuse problem, you have a one in four chance of developing that. Clinically and anecdotally it seems that once people have switched from misuse to abuse and to actually drinking to stave off the symptoms of withdrawal, it's better for them to stay abstinent. Then, we also need to treat the underlying behaviours or the problem in the first place: low self esteem, depression, anxiety, and looking at different coping strategies."

Trauma is something that emerges time and again in discussions on the cobweb of links between mental illness and addiction. A simple definition offered by Jane puts it that trauma occurs when someone has been subjected to an event where they thought they or someone else was going to die, and they felt helpless. This can result in post-traumatic stress disorder, where clients experience flashbacks, nightmares and poor sleep.

"When people have post-traumatic stress disorder there is a lot of activity in the fear system – the flight, flight, freeze or submit response – and their autonomic nervous system is highly raised. They can experience hypervigilance, sweating or avoidance behaviours," Jane says.

As Jo knows, trauma also impinges on addiction. According to Dr Ben Sessa, a consultant psychiatrist who specializes in substance misuse and psychopharmacology, it is the biggest single factor in the development of addiction.

"Addiction is a combination of psychosocial factors and physical effects on the brain, and of course, anyone can get addicted to a drug. Those of us who work with addicts see addiction in the medical model, as a disease. It is a complex disease, but all mental health problems are complex. The biggest factor is trauma: in many cases of addiction there is an underlying issue of trauma.

"Some of our patients may not have had 'Big-T' trauma – childhood physical or sexual abuse – but when we ask what their childhood was like, they may say, 'I never felt wanted, I felt neglected, I was never encouraged or praised, I always felt odd.' If a baby grows up in an environment that isn't safe, they develop an exaggerated amygdala response: everything is scary, they are always trying to avoid pain, there is hypervigilance. The more sophisticated prefrontal cortex part of the brain can normally overcome this amygdala response with reasoning and logic, for example, 'Well, it's not that bad, I can pull myself out of this.' But this can become a physical, hardwired brain change in infants, long before they get to any drugs.

"I always say to students, addiction is nothing to do with drugs: if you've grown up with trauma, you've got an addict's brain – a distorted reward–punishment system. When someone hands you a bottle of vodka at the age of 14, you're not scared for the first time in your life and you get a sense of reward and pleasure."

How alcohol affects the brain

Dr Ben Sessa: Alcohol has an inhibitor effect across all of the brain, dampening down cognition. It gives a sense of euphoria, which is why it is enjoyed, and has a very strong effect on the nucleus accumbens, which is the brain's reward centre where all drugs, from heroin to cocaine to cannabis, work. This is partly why it can become addictive. People who are heavy, dependent drinkers always score high on depression and anxiety symptoms, which is partly a pharmacological effect of the drug, and partly due to the damage associated with the lifestyle that comes with drinking.

Alcohol abuse and dependency

Using alcohol as self-medication is a slippery slope. Many people drink safely and benignly, but it's also a drug of abuse, which is why the government recognizes alcohol as a public health issue, with the guidelines of 14 units per week (seven pints of beer), for both men and women. Any more than that and someone would satisfy the diagnosis for harmful drinking.

In alcohol dependency someone is a daily drinker with much higher levels of intake. Alcohol has a strong physical dependence syndrome to it. Opiates (such as heroin), benzodiazepines and increasingly cannabis also have a strong physical syndrome. Cocaine has a strong *psychological* dependence, causing the desire to re-dose, without a particularly physical syndrome. In this respect alcohol is a nasty drug.

Physical dependence is dangerous because it is a depressant: if you use alcohol every day for weeks and suddenly stop, the brain is in a hyper-excited state, which can trigger seizure activity. If someone wants to stop drinking alcohol, they can either do it slowly and gradually, cutting down over weeks or months, or have a medically assisted detox, with high-dose benzodiazepines (lithium), primarily to protect the brain against seizure. Alcohol withdrawal also causes delirium tremens ("the DTs"): an organic psychosis that is a host of physical symptoms (sweating, diarrhoea, vomiting) plus the risk of seizure.

Alcohol & depression

It's difficult to accurately diagnose clinical depression in an alcoholic because we'd want to see what they're like without alcohol – in many cases when they stop drinking their mood improves. But there is a strong association between depression and alcohol, and depression and substance abuse can be tangled up in many ways.

Inasmuch as a person already has depression, they are more likely to turn to substances for self-medication. All substances have a positive euphoric effect at first, but it's not a very effective treatment. Secondly, there is the pharmacological effect of alcohol as a depressant and incorporated into that is the cycle of intoxication, withdrawal, craving, seeking and intoxication again. The other reason is that chronic alcohol misuse results in social deterioration: losing a job, family, kids, house and so on. These then become a risk factor for depression.

www.drsessa.com

Trauma, self-medication, addiction: when I think about this troubling trinity I remember what Sigmund Freud wrote about the escape from the "pressure of reality", and the search for "refuge in a world of our own". Life itself is traumatizing, and addiction can stem from the coping strategy that in the end proves dysfunctional – the cure that's as bad as the illness.

It also makes me think of another smart insight on drink and drugs, which I heard from Bez, the dancer from the famously hedonistic nineties band the Happy Mondays: "If you're doing it to celebrate, carry on. If you're doing it to hide: stop."

I'm in the "stopped" mode, and today as for tomorrow the challenge is to stay stopped, using methods that I've found to work. I guess that this talk of spiritual tools and higher powers can sound vague and strange, but what they come down to is a set of protocols for living sober and developing your life and yourself in the direction you'd like to see them go. So, I try to get through the day by practising gratitude, practising acceptance. Practising, full stop. Every day. (A gratitude list is another worthwhile addition to your story. Start itemizing the things you're grateful for, and add to it every day. Roof over your head and bed to sleep in? That's a good start).

But at the same time, I can reflect on what all of this spiritual home-work has done for me, and could probably do for you too. Mapping the stepwork, amending, listening and meditation onto "mental illness", it means that regardless of my personal configuration of depression, depend-ence and basic human despair, it doesn't matter whose "fault" any of it is. It won't help to blame the weather, the government, my hormones or upbringing, the unbelievable shit I've sometimes had to put up with, or the person who broke up with me or that filthy look the guy on the bus gave me last night.

It's up to me to make things right, live well and correctly and exercise what free will I have at my disposal to do so. And to realize that, in the grand and galactic scale of things, my suffering isn't any greater than anyone else's. Looking at things that way de-victimizes me. It's a strange kind of consolation, but it remains one nonetheless.

Did you stick with it? I hope so. It's been hard going because we've visited heaven and hell in this chapter, but I hope it hasn't sounded pious. Next it's time to get our feet back on the ground and go out into nature, at the same time as considering some more modern compulsions: technology, media and social media.

CHAPTER 8

NATURE & TECHNOLOGY

Green and screen in the recovery process and how one can solve the problem of the other: as with everything else, it's a matter of balance

In the water

Friday, late morning. Under a damp grey sky I'm standing on the jetty that extends into the middle of the Men's Pond at Highgate in north London, summoning the nerve to dive in. The water looks black, chilly and forbidding.

A few deep breaths as I reckon with it, making excuses. I adjust my goggles, fold forward and, with all the elegance of a sack of spuds falling off a lorry, plunge in.

The shock is total and instant, as if I've been electrocuted by adrenaline. A sudden wild euphoria.

Submerged, I thrash around in the bubbles, my breath held and skin tightening, then gather myself to the vertical and breach the surface, flipping onto my back and just floating for a while. I tread water as a duck paddles blithely past, then I stretch out and begin front-crawling toward the distant buoy.

I'm here with my friend David Baker, a journalist and broadcaster I've known and worked with since the late nineties. He's been in the water for some minutes now, serenely breaststroking the perimeter of the pond, perfectly comfortable under the overhanging boughs.

David is an all-year swimmer, coming here for daily dips in summer and autumn, and on through the winter and into spring, inured now to the chill and fortified by it. As for me, these occasional visits are somewhat conflicted: water isn't my natural element (I'm an Aries, a fire sign, in case you're into that sort of thing) and despite years of racing in triathlons, open water still gives me the shakes. Memories return of bombing into the deep end as a kid, and needing to be yanked out by the lifeguards. Ancient anxieties die hard.

On one of these visits David taught me an effective technique for dealing with water panic, when the muscles begin uncontrollably to tense, the heart rate soars and the breath quickens. He beckoned me over to a floating buoy, saying, "Look, focus on the moss here: the green turf on the white plastic hull. Make your looking continuous and microscopic, give it all your attention, and when the mind drifts off – to the fear of death by drowning, for instance – collapse it back to the object in front of you. Stay with it. Calm the breath."

It's a sort of mindful exercise in attentional control, and it works. My pulse slackens, my breathing stabilizes. I begin relaxing again. In swimming as in tai chi, everything improves when you relax.

So, this may be a conflicted experience, but these dips are stupendously revitalizing, a method for feeling instantaneously alive, anti-depressed; out of the water I find myself sprinting to the (even colder) showers, and notice the goosebumps on my arms and the muscles moving beneath skin.

But there's something else that makes these visits valuable, which is about direct experience: a purity of being that, for a moment, neutralizes all the cognitive interference and the ambient hassle of everyday living with its routines, schedules and transport connections, the needing to be somewhere or do something.

Compared with the sedentary fug of being at home or in an office, crackling with static and feeling mothballed, slightly too warm and a bit bored, this immersion in cold shocks me into a more vital bodily state, flatlining anxious worries and preoccupations. An experience of the material, elemental world as it is, in its raw, real self rather than its representation: water in its biting immensity, the moss and the duck close to me, and David in his total Davidness, bobbing in the water, chatting. So too is there a high-resolution experience of myself in all this: the chill penetrating my spine proves I'm alive.

This new state endures for a while. After we're done with swimming, we dry off in the changing area and make conversation with a few of the other men who frequent this most masculine of spaces. Idling awhile, I indulge in some diffident people-watching, studies in human zoology:

there are blokes holding yoga poses, others basking on towels, some quietly reading the paper, and still others parading impressive gym physiques – a Greco-Roman *tableau vivant* in leafy north London, 2019. Then David and I stroll off for coffee and a bun somewhere.

I notice myself just noticing all this, and this elemental experience is also singular: for a while I'm liberated from scrambled attention, the restless flitting between email and Facebook with the radio on in the background, my to-do list glowering at me on the desk, the marketing messages on the delivery van that just pulled up outside. I'm also released from the nagging feeling that while I'm doing one thing, I should be doing something else as well, such as washing the dishes while listening to the radio or eating lunch while I'm writing an email. Mono- instead of multitasking.

In swimming, I'm only swimming. I *can only* be swimming. Swimming is enough.

And lastly, I mean in the most basic terms that all this is an entirely unmediated experience: something done, felt, known and seen directly instead of through a browser window, a status update, in the pages of a magazine or in a video clip represented on the screen of a smartphone.

Media is the plural of *medium*, which can mean middle: the thing that *goes between* two other things. At the ponds there is no medium: nothing between me and the element of water, the duck or David. Life as real as life gets – at least until I decide to look at my iPhone.

Finding vitality

I wonder if you too enjoy moments like this – maybe in physical activity or in a certain location – where you feel vital, your experience of being alive stripped back to the essential, singular and simplified. Perhaps it comes in deep meditation, in dancing, singing, sex, involvement or movement, or watching a sunset, witnessing the frost on an extraordinary morning, or taking a long country walk into the dusk. And I wonder if you'd agree that these experiences can be like the exact opposite of the depressive state, where you feel zombie-like, alive yet somehow dead too.

I don't want to be too prescriptive here and suggest that a regime of chilly al fresco swims will instantly heal you (even though new evidence shows that cold-water swimming can assist with depression).[13] The point is these elemental experiences are worth making a habit of – literal "liveners" to the deadening and often sedative effects of technology.

I also hope that in this chapter I don't come across as a tinfoil-hatted Luddite, nor as some evangelist for the natural world. I'm not suggesting that we start ritually destroying iPads or putting a brick through Alexa or Siri in the belief that we can return to some pre-technological state. We can't, and I'll also resist lapsing into the romantic mode here, suggesting that nature herself is the bountiful provider of all answers to human misery (actually, being in nature can be quite boring. It's not always transcendent visions and sumptuous, life-affirming sunrises; nature also means decay, disease and cowpats).

But I do mean to say that in an increasingly digitized, artificial world there are benefits and disadvantages to both, and finding a balance on the axis between nature and the elements and technology, along with what it pipes our way, will advance us a bit further in our recovery. We increasingly live our lives online, connected to the grid yet disconnected from others. But we're not quite in *The Matrix* just yet.

We can start the investigation with what's in our pockets: the smartphone, which is for most of us the portal into the virtual and away from the elemental.

David has become something of an expert in this subject, and it often occupies our conversations when we meet. It might be ironic that for someone who commentates on the relationship between humans and technology – David works for *Wired* magazine and presents documentaries on Radio 4 – he hardly uses social media. He even – horror of horrors! – leaves his smartphone at home when he goes out for the day.

I compare this with my own smartphone use, and in doing so mine starts to look compulsive, if not exactly addictive. It's true that along with my laptop I'm dependent on it to the extent that I couldn't really do my work without it, but sometimes I resent the hold it has over me. I look at it first thing in the morning, switching between email, Facebook, Instagram and some news websites, aware all the while that I should probably be doing something more wholesome instead – getting outside for some fresh air, practising tai chi, eating some avocado on toast (I hate avocado). It's too much of a thrill to see if anyone has liked my Insta posts or the vlog

I uploaded to Facebook. Green-coloured notifications announcing the arrival of SMSs or WhatsApp messages are similarly pleasing. *I'm popular!*

Conversely, the absence of them can cause me to feel… what, exactly? Unloved? Un-approved-of? *Disliked*, even? When I look at it that way, the problem appears to be me and my emotions, rather than the smartphone itself. Which also means I can do something about it.

Still, this pattern tends to repeat throughout the day. I switch the phone off if I'm working on something that demands my complete attention (or if I'm sulking or suffering "phoneliness", convinced that no one likes me because the phone never rings), but I find myself compulsively fumbling for it when I'm on the train or waiting outside a café for someone to show up.

The notion of "smartphone addiction" has produced a number of sensational headlines recently, often centring on parental anxieties over the use of screens by young people and children: kids so entranced by, say, Snapchat or Fortnite that they never leave the sofa.

But what's the truth of it? Is smartphone addiction really a thing? And how does it relate, if at all, to the growth in reported rates of anxiety and depression in the last decade?

In 2018 David presented a fascinating Radio 4 documentary on all this (*Screens and Teens: Are Smartphones Harming Our Kids?*), and one of the featured speakers was Amy Orben, a psychologist at the University of Oxford who specializes in studying how social media shapes relationships and influences well-being. Wanting to know more about the science behind this subject, I went to meet Amy, and one of the first things she said was telling in itself: "I read a lot of literature on what people thought about televisions in the fifties and sixties when they came into homes," she says. "They felt quite similar to how we feel now." Bewildered, mystified and rather alarmed, probably.

Recently Amy has been involved in a number of public debates over claims around the negative effects of social media and screens. The argument is highly polarized: some researchers lobby for "screen time" to be limited; others say the available data doesn't back up claims that technology use is harmful to well-being, and this is Amy's view.

"We're still trying to figure it all out," she says. "We're at the very beginning. The public wants answers now, and we can't really give them."

Amid the fevered headlines, it's easy to forget that seemingly permanent and ubiquitous platforms such as Facebook and Instagram are relatively new, in historical terms at least. As are smartphones: I got my first mobile in 1999 and a Blackberry a decade later, by which time Facebook had migrated to mobile.

I'm also old enough to recall the first digital technologies, such as they were, arriving in schools. Installed into our third-year maths class in 1985, the primitive BBC Micro computer seemed like a mystical object, despite having all the presence and design flair of a breadbin. These machines were part of a larger project to enhance literacy, yet none of us was able to use them for anything more edifying than playing Snake for hours on end. At university a few years later, I was still writing my essays longhand, then keying them into a friend's electronic typewriter, which had an LCD screen the size of a matchbox. I'm a part of the generation that transitioned into the virtual new world, growing up as it accreted around us. The costly Apple laptop I'm writing this on may look and feel a bit nicer, but in absolute terms not much has changed. As for smartphones, mine still only rings when it wants to, as did the landline at my parents' house.

Amy tempers the debate around the presumed evils of "screen time", urging a more nuanced understanding.

"Screen time can be looking at your phone when you're setting your alarm clock or Skyping your grandma or scrolling through photos of Kim Kardashian. These all have very different effects. If we look at it so broadly, we'll never get a clear answer, so we're very far away from saying we're addicted to something. The term is misguided."

She adds that when it comes to a direct, causal relationship between technology and well-being, the data shows something – but that something isn't big enough to provide a clear answer.

"People have been finding this negative effect of technologies on well-being, and we do find them throughout the data sets, and they are negative, but they're extremely small. When we compare them to other activities that we've known for decades are important for our well-being – getting enough sleep and, for a child, eating breakfast before school – then technology's negative effect on well-being is a lot smaller than those effects, often up to three times smaller.

"So, should we invest billions into decreasing technology use, or should we invest time into making sure that people get enough sleep? We can't infer causality. These studies are mainly correlational, so we are looking at an association. It could well be that more technology use leads to lesser well-being, but it could well be that lesser well-being leads to more technology use."

Then there's the idea of "smartphone addiction". This too deserves scrutiny. Claims have been made that certain social media features – Facebook's Like button, notifications and the pull-to-refresh function on the app – stimulate a dopamine response, and scans of the brain prove it. The pleasure centres light up as they do when, say, a line of cocaine is ingested (in some cases, the developers responsible for these features have since denounced them for their addictivity.)

But it's all a question of degree, Orben says. "Our brains light up whenever we do something that's pleasurable, whether reading a newspaper, eating some pizza, doing drugs or using our phones. The comparison is valid, but it doesn't show that something's addicting – it shows that something's pleasurable to us. We never say that, Oh, reading a magazine is addicting because the same brain areas light up."

I have to say, too, that talk of smartphone addiction seems tendentious in the light of the struggles and sufferings of people I've known with genuine, life- and sanity-threatening dependencies to drink and drugs: conditions that all too often end in jails, institutions or death. I've seen friends quitting social media "for good" only to relapse a few months later, but it's difficult to view scrolling through kitten GIFs in the same light as chronic alcoholism or addiction to controlled substances.

Let's talk about loneliness

So I may not be a member of what's been called "iGen", the generation born after 1995 who have only ever known digital technology as a fixture of their everyday environment. But I doubt my psychological wiring is much different from theirs, nor very different from that of early humans who built the first technologies from wood and flint.

But what I have noticed in the last decade or so is a certain elusive erosion in the quality of social relations – I mean the web of friends, colleagues and family connections, the real-life interactions and the person-to-person, me-and-you meetings-up that merge into what we call "a social life". Much of it appears to have been supplanted by virtual connections: texts, chats and comments, and relations mediated by screens, profiles and emojis.

This, again, cuts both ways: I've both found and made friends through Facebook, Skyped people on the other side of the world and enjoyed the oceans of total and utter dross served up through pipework owned by the Big Tech unicorns: Twitter, LinkedIn, YouTube and so on. However, by the time I was fed up with living and working alone in London toward the end of the 2000s, my laptop seemed to have become my Significant Other – I was single, again, and many old friends were deep into the drift of cohabitation, marriage and family. Much of what made me want to decamp to Berlin was the prospect of finding new friendships IRL, and to sample the quality of social interaction in a city rather less nervous than London. I took my bike with me and rode around town, inviting myself to things, getting numbers, friending. Facebook helped. And it may seem grimly ironic that, in the absence of an ability to use my smartphone to actually speak to someone, its Facebook app was also where I posted my desperate "I need help" message five years later, almost to the day.

So it feels easy to blame digital technology, and smartphones in particular, for this decline in physical sociability, and it's especially easy to feel excommunicated from the entire human race when, upon entering a packed train carriage, we see literally everyone is glued to a screen with their headphones plugged in. My big fear – and perhaps it's a personal one – is that the forfeit made by the convenience of technology is to weaken something deep and tender within us: empathy, perhaps. The capacity to feel how someone else genuinely feels, the better to understand them. This is especially true with smartphones, which set up a primary physical choice between relating to it, or to an actual human. In my mind this is why therapy apps can only ever be partially effective. In therapy, as I said before, so much of the process is based on the literal, physical being with another person.

But regardless of the causes of what Orben calls "social fragmentation", it can produce a simple effect: loneliness, symbolized in the phone that stays obdurately silent, never ringing.

"What we've been seeing," she says, "is that in the last few years, people are feeling more connected but they're feeling more lonely, and naturally we don't have the scientific means yet to say something caused something, but the question is open."

Orben points out some further facets of this paradox of connection at the expense of isolation. She talks of the "Dunbar Number" (named after Orben's PhD tutor, Professor Robin Dunbar) of 150, which refers to the upper limit of stable social relations that a person can maintain. Many more than that, and we'd need a bigger brain.

"Why can we only have a certain number of friends?" Orben says. "Normally it's limited because of time: to have friends, I invest time in them and I need to remember all of their problems. It seems to be changing because on the one hand we don't really need to remember what people are doing any more. We have that on Facebook, and that is also decreasing the amount of time we need to connect with people. People feel drawn to the newsfeed, and I think that's because social information has always been key to how we survive. But we also know that social connection is more than just information transfer."

She means that all relationships are marked by a disclosure of selves to one another that happens gradually over time (or rapidly, in the event that you go to bed with them). The process of building trust. But the frames and filters of social media skew this yet again.

"We're losing this important reciprocal and balanced cycle of information transfer," Orben argues. "We don't know what the effect of that is, yet. We know that there are currently huge changes going on in the way social systems that have evolved over millions of years are functioning: we're still programmed to be our primate selves with the way we feel connected, but all of a sudden we're in a totally different social environment."

Talking to Amy makes me reflect on how I use social media, and though we didn't discuss three common psychological impulses that it seems to stimulate and even normalize – voyeurism, exhibitionism and narcissism – I can easily see them at play in my own social media habits. I notice myself becoming a voyeur when I'm bored, scrolling back through the feeds and looking at other people's wonderful holidays, relationships and parties. When I'm really bored, my inner exhibitionist comes out and

I start posting (what I like to think are) amusing photos, videos showing me cavorting around: attention-seeking, pure and simple.

However, I know I'm in trouble when I'm agonizing too much over a selfie or marvelling at how cool I look. Usually it's a sign that I'm basically very lonely, and I've been spending too much time alone. More broadly, narcissism seems to me a greater problem than the presumed addictivity of social media, since both on and offline it genuinely cuts us off from relationships with others.

As Amy says, it's not yet possible to say whether social media or the encroachment of digital technology is good, bad or indifferent for mental health.

"One person might be very positively affected by it, another person negatively. Some children are negatively affected, but it also allows people to connect with groups that they wouldn't normally reach out to. Children who've gone through a lot of trauma who Skype their friends, for example."

And for all the talk of Scroll Free September and digital detoxes, she adds that it's up to everyone to figure out the rules for themselves.

"A blanket approach telling people what to do won't work. Most people will be fine with technology: we can self-regulate. A lot of teenagers we talk to understand when they're doing too much and when their mood drops.

"I'd also say that people need to be more introspective and see what different kinds of technology affect them, and then try to maximize those that make them feel good. Things that connect us with people, where there's a direct cycle of communication, talking over FaceTime and messaging – those are all ways that we connect, socially."

Feelings have seasons

Technology, it seems to me, tends to atomize us into our own micro-worlds: the famous "filter bubble", which is echoed in the broader social trend toward individuation, of single occupancy, pursuing one's dreams and being a self-employed "entrepreneur" of the kind one sees a lot on Instagram.

There's another way, of course: just switch it all off. Cash in your smart-phone for a device that only does voice and text, and implement an ascetic rationing of Internet use by installing some browser blockers. These might help diminish all the competing thrills and aggravations of screen-based media, at the expense of a temporarily diminished sense of connection.

There is, naturally, a lot more opinion and advice online concerning the impact of technology and social media on mental health. In fact, there's no end of it, and trying to digest it all is likely to make you feel a bit... crazy. But to stay for a moment more with the uneasy relation-ship between screens, social media and depressive disorder in particular, something that made a lot of sense to me was a blog written by a friend of mine, Kati Krause, in 2015.

I'd got to know Kati soon after I moved to Berlin. Kati is a writer and editor, like me. As new friends and kindred spirits, we felt the urge to work on something together – a collaborative publishing project – and the cue came with the winter of 2012–2013, which, even by Berlin's extreme standards, was exceptionally bleak.

As usual the skies grew dark and the temperatures fell below zero sometime in late November 2012. They stayed that way well into the following April, and this brutally arctic season went down as one of the greyest on record, the sun hardly ever breaking through. In May it was common to see people emerging into the fresh sunlight looking profoundly haunted, as if returning from internment in a Siberian prison camp, with the pallor to match.

It certainly felt a bit chillier than usual. One evening I went for a run around the streets and upon returning home noticed icicles in my beard. I checked the temperature: it was −11°C.

Everyone was thoroughly depressed, ravaged by a city-wide pandemic of SAD (Seasonal Affective Disorder), and even the most emotionally buoyant Berliners could be seen staring at the pavement and reporting feelings of devastation and hopelessness. Luckily, the equally extreme Berlin summer, where the opposite usually happens, was just round the corner: in August and July I'd often find myself pinned to the sofa, utterly unable to move as the temperatures reached 39°C day after sweltering day.

This natural cycle of sunshine and greyness, warm sun to freezing fog, and our response to it as citizens of the biosphere, was what our magazine was about. It was entitled (of course) *Winter*, and along with our designer friend Ana Lessing, we commissioned a range of writers, artists, designers and photographers to make creative responses to this traumatizing meteorology: to get something of their experiences down on paper, out into the world and shareable. We completed the mag, launched a crowdfunding campaign, got it printed and then threw a cathartic launch party – a celebration of the joy and optimism that naturally follows bleakness and despair.

We may inhabit weatherless, temperature-controlled micro-environments (offices, supermarkets, shops and social spaces), but we're connected to the elements and the cycles of the seasons more deeply than we might guess. We're objects of the weather's own moods and nowhere is this more obvious than in the transition from autumn to winter when the clocks go back, the temperature drops and, often, our moods do the same.

Feelings are seasonal, and humans need fallow periods too.

As for Kati's blog (*Facebook*'s *Mental Health Problem*, @katikrause on medium.com), she posted it back when the debates over screen time and smartphone addiction weren't quite as shrill as they are today. And in it she talks about her decision, upon succumbing to a depressive episode, to delete all the social media apps on her phone, and then to log off from the sphere of social media completely (something I've noticed more and more friends doing recently).

Justly, her post went viral: it rang true, articulating something widely felt. It also offers a precise analysis of the antagonisms between social media (and Facebook in particular) and the experience of being depressed, which for Kati came down to three important insights. She wrote that in the midst of her depressive phase:

1. I wasn't able to perform for social media any more. I used to go through life mentally composing tweets and spotting photo opportunities for Instagram. That was unthinkable now. The mere thought caused so much anxiety that I could barely unclench my jaws.

2. I now consciously suffered from comparing my life to others', which was also new.

3. I was experiencing a powerful craving for instant gratification that also felt incredibly harmful... and wreaked further havoc on my already suffering attention span.

If you can recognize the impulse to compare and the craving for red-dot gratification above, I'm with you. But what powerfully told the truth for me was the first entry on Kati's list above, since it echoed something I'd wrestled with for a long time.

Recall what Dr Tim Cantopher said a few chapters ago about "avoiding any unnecessary challenges and only, where possible, doing what is easy." Among the biggest of these is a pressure to perform – to be a certain person – which for me had often meant constructing and maintaining a plausible and appealing image: as cool east-London DJ guy, and as focused, overachieving triathlete, for instance. Obeying this impulse was also what had made me feel uncomfortable when in my mid thirties I'd been working in the nattily suited men's magazine world, confecting myself as a witty and stylish man-about-town – but submerged beneath it, the fear that if I couldn't perform this role or wear this persona well enough, I was condemned to pity, and perhaps even scorn.

I'd tried to dismantle these images and wondered why we're urged to create "personal brands" in the first place. After all, personal brands won't be much use if the person behind the brand isn't functioning well, and feels deeply split, divided against themselves, as I often had. Point being, reading Kati's blog it struck me that social media is only, really, an exponential, multidimensional version of the same thing I'd experienced back in the inky world of magazines and the attendant circus of fashion parties and icily cool subcultures: a turbocharged new "panopticon" (as you may know, the panopticon was the eighteenth-century philosopher Jeremy Bentham's design for prisons, in which visibility – being seen – is what keeps prisoners under control, forcing them to conform). The difference is in extent and speed: there's way more social media where we're encouraged to be writer and editor in our own lives simultaneously. So too is it incessantly hungry, but it feeds on the same anxiety: Why am I afraid to tell you who I am?

We have the choice to engage with it or not, but the fundamental problem, it seems to me, is one of relating and the way in which this deathless pantomime of virtual performances transfers into actual person-to-person relationships. This is most obvious in the sphere of online dating, when images constructed online are exposed to the X-ray of "real" reality.

I dabbled with this in my mid-thirties and after a string of uneventful dates, it seemed to me that online dating was a great way for GSOH virtual profiles to meet each other (possibly more); it's rather less effective for humans in their complex, incoherent materiality. More often than not, it just made me feel astonishingly lonely.

Naturally, I gardened my profile such that I'd appear as what I imagined to be as attractive as possible: photos showing me looking slim, blazered and cheekboned, with text modestly alluding to my creativity and success in life, and self-deprecating remarks revealing me as a sensitive yet wordly man: "a catch". And no doubt the women whose profiles I Liked did the same.

My strategy was to bring these embryonic relationships into the three-dimensional reality as soon as possible, so that my date and I could begin to generate an accurate idea of one another, rather than relating purely as two images or "profiles", and begin the process of finding out each other's idiosyncrasies, emotional nuances, hopes and fears: basically, seeing if we fancied each other in 3D as well as 2D. This gradual self-disclosure is what actually constitutes a relationship, or in far less romantic terms, the "important reciprocal and balanced cycle of information transfer" Amy Orben talked about before. The being-with that staves off the chill of loneliness.

It never led to long-term love, mind. Done with online dating, my subsequent strategy was to launch myself into the human undergrowth in Berlin by simply going out, attending events, starting conversations and seeing where they went. Occasionally they went to Berghain, the famous Berlin nightclub. You may have heard that there's only one rule at Berghain: no photographs, which these days means no smartphones. Apart from that, you can do what you like, which means… well, you can probably imagine what it means.

Nor is any of this terribly new, even if it seems to be advancing at breakneck speed. Rather, it's the kind of thing French philosopher Guy Debord was talking about back in 1967 when in his work *The Society of the Spectacle* he wrote how "Everything that was directly lived has moved away into a representation." We needn't linger too long with Debord apart from to note that he predicted this massive and pervasive profusion of images, and the way in which this Piccadilly Circus-style "Spectacle" he conceptualized comes down to "a social relation among people, mediated by images." Meaning, when in real life I as Kevin-Profile relate to you as [Your Name]-Profile, the relationship is partial. Some important qualities – genuineness, our idiosyncrasies, that empathy I mentioned – seem absent.

If we're on any form of social media, we are mediating ourselves and observing others doing the same. On the other hand, relating directly rather than virtually, in person rather than through an image, is trickier and messier, with the risk of embarrassment and disappointment – but in the long term more fulfilling. I'm rarely stuck for friends to hang out with when I visit Berlin these days.

Still, what's the solution? One is immersion in the elements, a flight from the technological to the natural, the synthetic to the elemental and from mediated to direct experience. Going for a really long walk, for example.

Breaking the trance

Nature consoles and reduces, and contact with the elements imparts an almighty sense of littleness.

In his book *Wabi-Sabi For Artists, Designers, Poets and Philosophers* Leonard Koren wrote that truth comes from the observation of nature, and certainly nature offers simplicity in a demented world. However, we're less concerned with the "truth" here than with using what's around us to get or feel a bit better. Going into nature when the screens and media get a bit too much – when, for instance, you realize the only seashore you've seen recently has been on #Instagram.

From the nineteenth-century naturalist John Muir to more recent writers such as Robert Macfarlane, plenty has been written on the curative effect of nature on the emotional systems, and our increasing distance from it. Personally, I've also found solace in writers who use the world outside to explore the one within, such as Amy Liptrot in *The Outrun*, which tracks her recovery from alcoholism in the return she made to her native Orkney.

I was also struck by how in their book *Edgelands* the poets Paul Farley and Michael Symmons Roberts show the ways in which nature encroaches on our increasingly urbanized world. They advocate adventures into these "edgelands" – the light industrial zones and disused railway tracks where in summer butterflies congregate on buddleia and brambles sag with the weight of blackberries. This book returned me to memories of building dens with my friend Greg when we were kids, and also to my dad's copy of Richard Mabey's seminal book *Food For Free*, back when "foraging" wasn't quite the lifestyle trend it is today. Elderflower fritters weren't uncommon at teatime in our house.

There's nature, and there are the elements, and those are what I felt an urge for in 2014, a month or so after being taken to hospital in Berlin, when, back in the UK, I set off to walk the Offa's Dyke Path. Contact with the wild edges of the hard physical world at a time when the tangled circuitry of the psychological and emotional world had become too much.

One day in September I set off on the 177 mile route from Prestatyn on the coast of North Wales along the old border of England and Wales to Sedbury on the Bristol Channel, over mountains and valleys, along paths and lanes, beside streams and endless expanses of heather. It took about two weeks, with a few days off in the middle to give the blisters time to heal.

Walking is as much mood as activity, a way of being mindful without having to do mindfulness, and I noticed some of my agonies becoming digested through perambulation. Up in the gods and under the skies I recognized how loneliness can transform into solitude: when you're totally alone, nothing is missing or absent. Then one late afternoon, idling on a riverbank and spotting a kingfisher speeding past, it occurred to me that nature is the ultimate cinema, so long as you've got the patience for it. At the end of each day I turned my smartphone back on, sent a few texts, looked at Facebook and some headlines for a while, then switched it off, and began cleaning the dried mud off my boots.

Walking works, for me at least, as do those expeditions to the ponds with David and, when it's pouring down with rain, going for a run in the spirit of Cassius in Shakespeare's *Julius Caesar*: "And when the cross blue lightning seemed to open/the breast of heaven, I did present myself/Even in the aim and very flash of it". Most recently there's been gardening.

Early in 2018, I noticed that my mood had again sunk and obstinately refused to lift; I felt flatly depressed and pessimistic, cooped-up and cabin-feverish. There were some obvious causes – a bereavement, the grind of an endless winter and the fact that I was flat broke – but an answer to this perpetual bleakness was visible through my bedroom window. The back garden behind my flat, shared by the other resident in this property, hadn't seen the sharp edge of a spade for a long time. So I got stuck in, raking up leaves, extending a makeshift patio, digging a veg patch and laying a path from broken paving stones, then warming my hands in the unloved chimenea in the afternoons.

Sweat (water), mud (earth), swearing (air), fire (chimenea) and wood (everything else): all five elements in one therapeutic exercise. When spring finally arrived, I began to feel a bit better: digging against depression had done the trick. Give it a try.

The elements

There are only five. Here are a few ideas on embracing each one:

Air: get up high – a hill, vantage point, office block, or the highest point where you live – and get some breeze into the system. Failing that, be outside, practise breathwork and some cathartic yelling: scream your head off at a passing train or into a pillow. Singing and speaking also help.

Earth: walk, and notice the ground beneath your feet. Ideally, walk with no destination – we're not trying to "get" anywhere. The walking is the thing, not the completing, the speed, distance or the sights along the way.

Water: find a large body of it – pool, lido, river, lake, sea – and plunge yourself into it (but take precautions: go with a friend, don't go in if it's too cold or choppy, don't stay in too long). Alternatively, try a cold shower, a couple of hours in the sauna, or just sweat. If it's pouring down with rain go out for a walk, but rather than hiding in a protective waterproof shell, come home only when you're wet through.

Fire: build one, outside somewhere. You don't need firelighters, just paper, twigs, dry sticks, logs and then a match or a lighter, in that order. Ask permission and keep a bucket of water nearby. Note: green things don't burn. Fires are what we gather round, and collective experiences can stand in for them: a concert, mass gathering, demonstration, screening, barbecue, or a dinner you cook and host for friends.

Wood: take a day out somewhere wild and wooded for the absorption in deep greens and browns, observing the passivity of plants. Watch how they don't strain. Whenever you pass a florist or garden centre, make a point of calling in to inhale deeply.

CHAPTER 9

WORK & PURPOSE

Making money and making meaning, and how both can help

Another Friday morning, this time in Berlin.
The tram I'm on snakes its way along Greifswalder Strasse, one of the spacious arterial boulevards that radiate north and east from Alexanderplatz, which is the interchange of today's short journey.

Maybe you know "Alex", as it's called here, with the enormous *Fernsehturm* (TV Tower) in the middle, silently watching over the German capital. On bright days the shape of a crucifix can be seen on the steel exterior of the tower's immense orb, cast by the sun. Back in the communist era the authorities were enraged by this architectural quirk: Soviet rule had tried to eliminate religion from the world, but Berliners called this shadow "the Pope's Revenge", mocking the vanity of autocrats. Stories of division and trauma everywhere in this city – so too the presence of angels.

As the tram shudders to an abrupt halt I lurch into a handrail: we've stopped between two buildings. To the right is a solemn edifice that once housed the offices of Erich Honecker, leader of the German Democratic Republic until 1989. To the left is another mutely imposing structure, the Soviet-era *Haus des Reisens* ("House of Travel"). Formerly a collection of GDR travel agencies and visa offices, today it is occupied by a gym, a second-hand clothes shop and offices. There's a nightclub on the twelfth floor and another in the basement.

I know this place. It's familiar, and painfully so. We were here at the start of this book, the place where I hit rock bottom in 2014.

Peering through the tram windows, I see the rear entrance of the tower block leading onto an anonymous plaza: a bike rack, some people smoking, a set of steps. I remember exiting those doors a few years ago and then slumping down on those steps, helpless and saturated in tears. I was there for some time, consumed with what I now know is called suicidal ideation: an overwhelming urge to meet the end. Ideation turned into intention, thinking into doing, and then, after some time, the plea for help.

I'll never know how long I was there for, with the TV Tower winking at me from on high, the blinding August sun behind it.

That was 2014 and I've since been back to Berlin quite often, to retrace steps and see friends. This morning I'm on the way to meet my friend Enver. We're doing some more work together, making some more publications. I'm running late for our meeting but in any case, I don't care to linger at this spot even if in the intervening years it's been good to pass by and recollect occasionally, little by little effecting a gradual separation, and building a new relationship with this city and my pals here. This tram ride finds me between two buildings and two eras, perhaps even two lives.

Soon we move on through the traffic lights into Alexanderplatz and I stare up to the corner office on the fourteenth floor where in 2012 I started work as editor-in-chief. I lasted two and a half years and I remember the stresses it caused and how in the end they contributed to the crisis. Something that, in the world of work these days, would be written up as "a burnout" (as we know, the terminology is always approximate).

Just as I'm hastening to meet Enver, our enquiry needs to progress. In this chapter we'll look at work a bit more closely, considering some ways in which it can contribute to mental health (it can) as well as mental illness, and a bigger question that sits behind it: *what am I supposed to do with my life?*

The joys and sorrows of work (mainly sorrows)

Pain has no memory, thankfully. But when I contemplate the dynamics in play in that toxic job, some obvious stressors emerge, and I dare say some will sound familiar to anyone in a white-collar job in the corporate or creative sector.

My own over-involvement with the job was one thing: working as if my identity depended on it, or as if everything that went wrong was my fault, animated perhaps by low self-esteem. There was also the status that this position conferred on me while also entrapping me: being a magazine editor certainly helped me to get onto guest lists for nightclubs and fashion events, but the accompanying lonely-at-the-top feeling was acute – a shade of loneliness markedly different to the one I'd known as a freelancer. Worry and insecurity had been the norm as I subsisted on a pattern of feast-or-famine piecework: tons of work for a month, nothing for the next, meaning a complete inability to plan financially, and the sense that I was only ever as good as my last invoice. This latest employment brought a new dimension of anxiety.

In the daily work of managing writers, designers, photographers and stylists there was the need to phase between acting as a facilitator one moment (creative people often do their best work when they're most free), disciplinarian the next (deadlines need to be met) and a counsellor in between, offering tissues and sympathy when staff burst into tears due to, say, the latest unreasonable demand from the publisher or a long-overdue unpaid invoice.

Beneath all this sat something universal for those of us who belong to the economic 99 per cent: the primary need to hold down the job to make the money to put bread on the table. I remember something my friend Dawood (Chapter 5: Learning & Listening) told me a decade ago, when I was interviewing "youngers" involved in gang crime in south London. "The reality of these people's lives is that they have to *get money* every day," he said.

Money talks a language we all have to listen to: whether we're street-level dealers or high-powered execs on the corporate ladder, we're all hustlers involved in the daily matrix of compromises in what needs to be done to get paid. It may also be historically unprecedented how these days we look to work to provide something beyond mere remuneration, ideas such as purpose, fulfilment and satisfaction. Either way, in this job I remember that those were few and far between.

And by the way, working as a magazine editor isn't quite the jet-setting, power-lunching role it's often depicted as. The hard work, long hours and manic firefighting may have been making someone, somewhere, fulfilled or wealthy, but it definitely wasn't me. The truth was far more prosaic and routine: every day I'd cycle into work, chain my bike up, smoke a cigarette, then check in with the editors and designers, argue with the ad sales guy, curse the photocopier and set about deciding which on the long list of problems needed fixing most urgently. Often, I'd be emotionally shattered by lunchtime. I'd open the windows and take a breather, gazing north-east over Erich Honecker's office to the spires of Prenzlauer Berg, wondering quite how I got here, and whether it was all worth it.

Stress can be defined as what results when demands are made on a person who doesn't have the resources to meet them. Sound plausible? It did to me. Leaving work in the evenings, dazed and wired, I'd often slope off into the streets of Kreuzberg or Mitte, never quite knowing how to handle these conflicts or who to talk to about them. I'd then engage in the orthodox Anglo-Saxon approach to dealing with anguish: drowning it in drink.

A creeping sense of pointlessness in the endeavour bled into something else toward the end of my tenure in the job: an overcast in mood often so subtle I barely noticed it, like curtains gradually closing over my inner perceptual world, my sense of who I was. Stress, doubt and disorientation condensed into what we'd describe as depression; the decline into crisis was steep and rapid, but I was deaf to the signals.

Work, then: status at the cost of loneliness, a pay packet as the price of purposelessness and self-advancement at the expense of relationships because it's hard to climb the greasy pole by being nice, after all: these seem common dysfunctions today, when work is at its worst.

The upside is that if they do become too much to bear, perhaps it's the market's way of telling you that you're in the wrong job, or doing the wrong thing.

Mental health at work

It used to be common to see a jokey sign hung in offices with the side-splitting gag, "You don't have to be mad to work here, but it helps". Given the toxicity of many workplaces today, it probably needs modernizing: "You don't have to be mad to work here, but you soon will be."

The good news is that mental health in the workplace is a big issue these days, with campaigns and initiatives popping up in many offices and other workplaces. Perhaps where you work you've noticed managers or executives busily leading the charge to make workplaces more mentally healthy, offering access to counselling services, courses on mindfulness, resilience and mental health first aid, plus flexible working arrangements and campaigns to end the stigma attached to talking about illness, with the presence of workplace mentors, advocates and champions.

And not a moment too soon: to put it bluntly, work often seems to make people depressed and anxious, often intolerably so, and these days I know I'm hardly alone with the torments involved in trying to turn a penny. A 2017 survey by the City Mental Health Alliance of employees in law, insurance and banking said that 47 per cent had had experience of mental health problems in their current employment.[14] Another UK government report from 2017 showed that 300,000 people with a long-term mental health problem lose their jobs each year, and at a much higher rate than those with physical health conditions.[15]

Recent years have seen a number of suicides in the famously high-pressured financial sector of the UK, but the figures are yet more alarming at the other end of the income scale. In 2017 the Office for National Statistics reported that in the construction industry between 2011 and 2014 there were 1,400 suicides.[16]

If that sounds scandalous, there's one more statistic to mention here, which suggests that poor mental health costs the economy between £74 billion and £99 billion per year. To which we might easily respond: so what? What does it really matter if the UK, say, is less internationally competitive when you or I are racked with fear and despair on the daily commute? One needn't be a Marxist to wonder how much the economy really cares about our well-being so long as we're obediently creating value and consuming products.

Similarly, it's hard to look at the economic challenges faced by many people today, but especially the young – greater job insecurity, wider income inequality, zero-hours contracts, rising personal debt, often from tuition fees, declining social mobility and the lockout on home owner-ship – without wondering if the reported generational rise in depression and anxiety is simply the understandable response to living under the iniquities of a relentless market economy.

It won't help to get too polemic or political when we're thinking about the personal in the economic and what it means for recovery. But since we're talking shop let's at least be businesslike and ask: is the new emphasis on well-being at work, which is proven to enhance productivity, genuinely well intentioned, or simply a disguised effort to shore up the bottom line? Should companies really be interested in their workers' happiness, or is it purely a matter of personal responsibility? What to do when the "work" in the (somewhat idealistic) notion of "work–life balance" is the problem? And lastly, is the new business mantra of "bringing your whole self to work" – meaning, your wonky and splendid entirety – realistic, or just a fantasy?

"The last one sounds slightly utopian," says Georgie Mack, who among other things happens to be my boss from the most recent job I had.

Back to work after a burnout

Georgie is managing partner of a digital consultancy in London, and I met her in 2015 after applying for a job there. I'd seen an ad online and speculated that using my experience in editorial work might be beneficial, involving me in a sphere of activity outside the loop of my own thoughts. I liked the idea of going back to work after a year off. Plus, I needed to make some money.

I started work as an "embedded storyteller" in September that year, helping the staff at this company publish stories about what it does. I soon overheard that Georgie had begun running a series of mental-health-at-work meetups in the office. One day I mentioned to her that I'd had problems, and asked her if I could get involved, helping out with building a website, publishing blogs and so on, on a voluntary basis. Doing service, I remembered from my friends in the fellowships, was another proven method of getting or staying well.

The organization Georgie founded is called Minds@Work (www.mindsatworkmovement.com), and it has grown into a network of over 1,000 businesspeople, clinicians, coaches and innovators, all dedicated to eliminating the stigma that surrounds mental health and illness in the workplace. Its mission is to encourage business leaders to tell stories about their own mental health challenges, and in so doing mandate those difficult-to-have conversations throughout their companies.

Minds@Work began when Georgie teamed up with a friend of hers, Geoff McDonald, a gregarious South African who was vice president of human resources at Unilever, the transnational company that employs 170,000 people and makes consumer goods from Bovril to Brylcreem. Geoff is a big-business guy with a big network and a booming voice, but this dry character sketch doesn't do him justice: some years ago, as high up the corporate scaffolding as it's possible to get, he began suffering panic attacks and was diagnosed with anxiety-related depression. Not long after, a close friend of Geoff's ended his own life. These events effected a drastic reorientation in Geoff's life, and in recent years he has emerged as one of the leading champions of mental health at work, with the ear of industry titans, news media and politicians alike.

As for me, I didn't expect to return to work after more than a year out to meet others who'd had experiences of depression, anxiety, panic attacks and burnout, but so it proved. There are a lot of us about these days, as the subject itself creeps out from behind the therapist's couch.

Given all of this, Georgie has an acute view of the issues connecting work and wellness, and how poor leadership can both enhance and impede the latter. In the early 2010s when she was researching mental health for a design brief, she was alerted to something that an academic she interviewed called "an absolute looming crisis".

"I was absolutely appalled at how massive the numbers of people suffering were, and I was determined to try and do something about it," Georgie says.

Her interest isn't only professional; Georgie talks about how, in her twenties, she also suffered panic attacks so severe that she was unable to take a train or even go to the cinema. She devised her own coping mechanisms and eventually she was able to pull through.

"My hypothesis was that there is a universe of people who are in the early stages of mental illness," she says. "Most of them will create workarounds like I did but some of them won't. And when you fall, as we know, the climb back up is massive. It's a huge challenge." She means the kind of slide into crisis that I'd been through, along with others she's seen.

"It would be incredibly powerful if through the workplace we could get to people who might be having panic attacks, an uneasy relationship with alcohol, insomnia, feeling blue every day without knowing why: indicators of potentially larger problems."

Minds@Work isn't the only organization attempting to dismantle the stigma relating to mental illness at work, but it has been singularly successful in getting bigwigs to speak out, people for whom status in the hierarchy can count for a lot, and upon whose decisions the well-being of a company and its employees can rest.

If someone is in a very senior position and wields great power, if they speak out about mental illness, it can be transformative within an organization, Georgie says. "But if services, interventions and programmes are put in without leadership authentically embracing it, they will always fall short of their potential and impair people in coming forward. In places where leadership will not authentically say that mental health matters and make themselves vulnerable in front of their organization, then the employees will probably feel very challenged in being honest."

This stigma is real when, in organizations with pecking orders and office politics – that is, practically all organizations – status is hard-won and easily lost, a force that invisibly regulates the inner psyche of every company. In this respect, something that happened in 2017 is illuminating.

You may remember the email exchange circulated on social media in which manager Ben Congleton of the software company Olark commended an employee, Madalyn Parker, for her decision to take a day off to prioritize her mental health; doing so was totally cool by him. The exchange quickly went viral as an example of enlightened leadership in the age of anxiety.

Yet it probably shouldn't be news, particularly if as employees and employers we're serious about the "parity of esteem" between mental and physical health that was announced by the UK's coalition government in 2013. At the same time, many workplaces today may not be so understanding. It's easy to imagine that behind such a heart-warming tale are many more examples of workers attracting opprobrium and even losing jobs as a result of confessing to experiencing difficulties, diagnosed or otherwise.

Either way, as Georgie sees it, "There's a huge way to go in the business world. One thing people often say is that mental health is 50 years behind physical health in terms of how we think about it and the treatments available, and it's well understood that depression will be the global disease of burden by 2030. We will have to do some massive leapfrogging."

Mental health is on the workplace agenda and is, correctly, seen as more than an adjunct to corporate social responsibility programmes. "Some organizations now have a higher-order purpose that they live and breathe," Georgie says. "They put people front and centre, and that attitude is designed into every part of how they operate. The same will happen with employee mental health and well-being: really good organizations will future-proof themselves, design themselves to bring out the best in their employees, in the way the space is designed, the services that are available, people are incentivized."

But we're not quite there yet. "There's a lot of noise, and we haven't quite knocked the stigma down. It's brilliant when an organization is trying to do something, even if it's driven by pure economics and not ethics. But there's a lot of box-ticking going on; if organizations honestly think that sending a few people on a mental health first-aid training makes a difference, think again."

One way to test this is, of course, to "phone in mad" one day, and see how your manager reacts. While I was working for Georgie, there was at least one day when I had to. Waking up with a nameless, causeless despair, I reasoned that "my whole self" was better off staying in bed rather than imposing it upon work and glumly presenteering for the day. I texted Georgie and her colleague Charlotte, who was in charge of human resources. To my immense relief it was fine by them – a response that wasn't necessarily worthy of going viral but was simply an example of empathy in action. I was lucky to have such an empathic employer, and the scenario also seemed a world away from my job in Berlin, where I had the feeling that pleas for help, on my part and all the way up to my former boss, would fall on deaf ears. Companies may be waking up to the need to take mental health seriously, but again, there's a long way to go.

"Employers do have a responsibility to their employees to look after their mental health and well-being within the workplace as far as they are able," Georgie says, "Because quite often it is the conditions of the workplace that can exacerbate or catalyze mental ill-health within employees."

Meanwhile, it's one thing to be an employee struggling at work and knowing what do to about it: asking for help is a good way to start. But it's another thing to be in the other role: a manager of people, any of whom might be suffering in silence. This again can be tricky terrain in the landscape of modern business, with genuine cases of mental illness dismissed or overlooked.

Georgie is similarly decided on this too: "Employers also have a massive responsibility to make anyone who is a line manager as well equipped as possible to deal with people who report in to them, not just within the context of work, but thinking about their well-being more holistically."

The art of managing well comes down to one thing, Georgie argues. "However much we try to codify ways of behaving, every human being and every context is unique: there'll never be an exact step-by-step solution. But as long as you, as a manager, are compassionate, empathic, and you listen, you won't go terribly wrong. Hanging on to humanity is absolutely key." Carl Rogers would certainly have approved, and probably agreed that it's good to get back to work.

It felt that way in late 2015 when, with my pencils sharpened and specs polished, I started this job, looking forward to being productive again. It worked so long as I was honest with myself and others, even if the process was often fretful, with days when I was inwardly gripped with worry and self-doubt (could I really do this job, was I liked, would my work make any difference?). "Worked" as in: helped me function, gave me the chance to contribute and serve and offered some new and nourishing friendships. It was also a job I could leave at the gates every evening, as all jobs ought to be.

Calling in for a meeting one afternoon, Geoff McDonald took me aside and renewed his insistence that returning to work is good for recovery: it's a way of being purposeful and interacting with others. It gets you involved in something bigger than yourself, and reminds you of what you're good at, or at least what you can do.

The burden of purpose

The nature of work is changing today, and given that most of us spend 40 hours per week doing it, this naturally has an effect on how we think and feel about ourselves. Some of the contingent factors are listed above (greater insecurity, zero-hours contracts and so on) but there are plenty more, often driven by technology. We hear a lot about how an increasingly digitized economy promises a liberation from manual work and how in the future robots will do all the labour. There will, it's said, be greater flexibility in the form and rhythm of work, with the possibility, for instance, of being a "digital nomad" working wherever in the world has decent Wi-Fi or 4G. For a moment let's set aside the fact that the wealth created in these new sectors tends to trickle upward to a tiny elite of Silicon Valley billionaires. Instead let's ask what this means in relation to the question this chapter started with: what am I supposed to do with my life?

For a start, it's interesting talking to Georgie about the common aspirations of the type of person her company often recruits: so-called millennials, digital natives and Generation Z-ers who enter the workforce with very different ideas to the ones I entered with, and ideas totally foreign to those shared by my parents and their parents, who were all factory workers. Georgie observes how these days people don't want jobs that "just look good, but feel good too": pleasant workspaces with free amenities from expensive craft coffee to on-the-job learning and extended parental leave.

At the same time work and "life" (meaning leisure time, relationships, the stuff we do for fun) often collapse into one another. The overspill can be one of the contributory factors in mental illness, when the aggravations of the working day are taken into evenings and weekends. But here Georgie means how it is becoming rarer to follow the linear post-war path from education to work to family to more work to a retirement based around gin, tonic and cruises on the Med. In its place she perceives the desire for "a dissolving between work and travel and learning", ambitions to "feel some pride in what the organization they're working for represents and what they're doing in the world" (acting ethically as corporations) and alongside that "a need for people to express themselves over and above just the workplace."

These are, of course, admirable aspirations and incredibly attractive, too: who wouldn't want a job where an employer allows you to write code on a Thai beach before putting in some voluntary hours at the nearby wildlife sanctuary and then working on your creative side-hustle, perhaps over a few sundowners adjacent to the moonlight rave? It sounds awesome, and social media tells me that a deficit of awesomeness in one's life may result in a terrible case of FOMO (the fear of missing out).

❧

Yet as far back as 1943 the American psychologist Abraham Maslow pointed out in his well-known "hierarchy of needs" that stable human functioning relies on some very basic needs (food, water, shelter, security, belonging) being met before these higher-order aspirations (pursuing a goal, finding happiness) can be fulfilled. These tend to be contained in the fashionable idea of "purpose", which is another thing we're all supposed to have these days. But I often wonder what it means for the soggy Deliveroo rider who bravely cycles up to my flat against a brutal headwind to deliver pizza on a dark Thursday night. I speculate that an overgenerous tip might assist, at least, with some of his more basic Maslowian needs, such as rent, if not the need that is closely associated with depression: esteem.

I mean to say here that the tension in day-to-day life between what you need to get (recall my friend Dawood and his youngers) and what you want to do, like those Gen-Z digital nomads, is what our enquiry is about because so much of it impinges on notions of identity and capability, which often come unstuck in experiences of mental illness and health. Questions such as Who am I? What is the point of today? And What is the meaning of life? arise as gigantically unanswerable thought-bubbles.

The notion of an overarching, self-defined "purpose" that suffuses one's life with shape and direction... well, it's reassuring to believe that this will offer a reply to those questions, yet it could just as easily be another burden – a prescribed need, and something liable to prompt anxiety if you can't find one or can't enact it, or if this divine purpose doesn't pay the bills. Like vulnerability, passion and authenticity, purpose makes for a good hashtag, and while we may all want to give back, make a difference and save the world in whichever way we can, the world (and the market) usually has its own ideas.

Looking back at the 25 years I've spent working, I can see how I've navigated this tension at times deftly and at other times dumbly. Being a writer may be a creative profession, and creativity is often considered to be more nourishing for the soul. But work is paid by the word and the story, so no words or stories, no pay. My career, such as it is, has also been haphazard, a combination of application and aptitude along with a lot of being in the right place at the right time: what's known as luck. But there's something else: the times when I've felt I've been most creative, resolved and satisfied are usually the times when I've been poorest and most financially precarious. Similarly, when I've been lucky enough to be offered well-paid but uninspiring work, the pocket money may have kept me warm at night, but it did little for the condition of my soul. After two and a half decades, the trade-off seems clear.

In this I've veered between two poles typified in the archetypes of the artist and the banker: the former works in their garret to faithfully bring a tortured but highly authentic vision into reality, at the expense of financial and social success; the latter is concerned with the management and accrual of cash with a cost, perhaps, of a certain spiritual emptiness. The artist envies the banker for his or her comfort and affluence, the banker envies the artist for their creativity and aliveness to the aesthetic world. One rarely hears of poor but fulfilled bankers, or wealthy and comfortable artists.

Above all, this seems to be the compromise we need to strike between making money and making the meaning that all lives need – and meaning is the thing that stands behind the sacred new creed known as purpose. Meaning – the "why to live" – is what Viktor E. Frankl, who we met in Chapter 4, said we can all make.

So, if you're struggling, perhaps give the search for purpose a miss for now. For one thing, a rock-bottom moment is a sure sign that you cannot keep on with whatever it was that dragged you down, whether a toxic habit, relationship or job. But instead of busying yourself to discover a whole new direction in life today, how about making recovery your new and absorbing purpose?

Work it – boss it, even – and it may prove to be the most creative and fulfilling thing you ever do even if, or perhaps directly because, no one is paying you to do it. Your life's purpose, assuming it needs one, will find you when it will. Plus, what you learn along the way might help others too. That's something to think about for your story.

Speaking of stories, here's the final one for this chapter. I left the job that Georgie had given me in the autumn of 2017, after two years in the role. My mum had become ill and I needed to spend time with her, and alongside that my *Torchlight* project had suddenly taken off: an article I wrote about it for the *Observer* newspaper went viral, and everything Enver and I had made sold out. Suddenly, a new vocation had found me.

But in a roundabout way all this too had come from the job at Georgie's company. Its title, as I said, was "embedded storyteller", which initially sounded a bit fantastical to me. Nevertheless, it made me think I'd better start telling some stories. So, in the evenings and weekends I also started writing down the details of what had happened to me in Berlin, what went before and what happened after; the text that turned into our *Torchlight* publication.

Like love, purpose is something that finds you when you're least looking for it.

Back to the project of getting better: very soon we'll talk about ways to start work and keep the work up with the idea of "practice": the stuff you do every day to get better. Before we do, though, there's one more subject to address.

CHAPTER 10

TO PARENTS

Some thoughts for parents of children of any age who are suffering, and for children if and when their thoughts turn to their parents. Plus, the subject of love.

I hope that by now it comes through clearly that this story of recovery has involved a lot of people, and plenty of experiments. In the months and years that followed my slide into crisis in Berlin there were sudden accelerations in the course of getting or feeling better, with minor and modest miracles. There were also false starts and plenty of setbacks that arose seemingly from nowhere – days or weeks where I simply felt lifeless, as if nothing that I could do or had done would make any difference. Trial and error, and dead time filled with dead feeling. These phases remain in my life, but these days they're less frequent, and rarely last long.

The only real constant throughout all this was people: the ones who were present (calling, visiting, offering a place to stay and a chance to hang out) and the ones I made the effort to see, and then the people who, like those setbacks, appeared as if from nowhere to offer a helping hand or some wise words, totally unbidden. This is why in this book I talk a lot about what I've learned from friends and people I've met.

But there are some people I haven't really mentioned until now and who are perhaps conspicuous by their absence: my parents; and here I want to say something about them, along with something else that's important in the recovery process: love, and making the decision to always try to love others, oneself and life itself too.

A telephone call

It was a Wednesday when the phone rang and when it did it showed my sister's number, but it was my dad's voice on the line. I knew what this meant, and I was at Cannon Street station when the meaning arrived. It was November 2017 and the sky was white.

It meant a prognosis – a time frame. We'd been needing one. "We" being my mum, dad, sister and me, and then the concentric rings of family, friends and others radiating around from our immediate, embattled unit. It meant the time the doctors reckoned my mum had left, meaning also the time we had with her. She'd been ill with cancer for the previous 18 months: contracted and overcome it only for it to return pitilessly, yellowing her skin to the colour of sand. Breast cancer to begin with, and now cancer of the organs.

She'd had a big operation and the surgeons had removed part of her stomach – apparently people can live without a stomach, I never knew this – but the medics couldn't remove all of what they referred to as the "structures". Tumours, the hidden malignancies. After months of waiting and following Mum around as she was shipped from ward to ward, hospital to hospital, back home and out again, beds, scans, ambulances and elevators – well, now we knew.

Leaving Mum in her bed on the ward every evening, with her books and her headphones, was very hard to do.

That Wednesday I dried my eyes and moved around London, doing the usual stuff I have to do, but I screwed up the journey back to my flat, and ended up waiting for ages at Clapham Junction at rush hour. I felt incredibly sad – absolutely voided, in truth. I got back home and rang Mum, reassuring her that we'd all be around, just to love her right until this end that we now knew was going to happen, and then far beyond. All the way, Mum.

I told her about all the texts and messages of love and support that I'd been receiving, destined for her, from friends all over the place – Berlin, France, the US and Down Under, people she knew and others she'd never heard of, and these messages moved her. I told her that I loved her and that she was the best mum in the world ever.

It was pitch black that November night, and sitting at the window of my bedroom I wrote a list of things I wanted to say to her and ask – final conversations – and the next day I took this piece of paper up north to the house she'd lived in with my dad for decades, the one where my sister and I had grown up.

I'd been making this long and empty journey for many months now, often twice a week; door to door it was five hours and as many trains away from my flat in south London, with a lonely walk along country lanes at the other end. New Cross Gate, London Bridge, Euston, Birmingham International, Shrewsbury, Gobowen; me and my bag, boots and Barbour jacket against the wind and drizzle. Mum used to pick me up in the car when I visited at weekends, and only some way into this new pattern did I realize that it would never happen again.

The things you realize when someone's dying or has died – things ended, things gone and gone forever. The final text message she sent me was: "Xxxxxxxxxxxxxx from Mum".

I don't know if the doctors actually used the word "prognosis", or if it's still part of the oncology vernacular these days, but the prognosis, Dad had told me, was weeks. And it was exactly weeks, no more or less: two weeks. Mum died a fortnight later, peacefully in a hospice around 9 p.m. The Wednesday after the Wednesday after that Wednesday when Dad rang on my sister's phone to break the news, as I was getting off a train at Cannon Street, pausing, swamped by the sorrow of life, and wondering what the f*** to do.

Since that call I'd camped at my parents' house. I was there for the foreseeable. Talking to Mum, bringing her things, arranging her pillows, comforting her, then staring into space in the adjacent bedroom when she was asleep. I helped her up when a few days later the paramedics came to put her in the ambulance to the hospice. I held her upright while she collected some things in her bag and then off to the hospice, where she slipped into the mercy of a wakeless sleep, the leaves on the birch trees through the windows turning shades of amber, robins and wagtails pecking around.

One day my sister said, "It won't be long now," (my sister is a GP) and so it proved. The hospice was half an hour from our house, and my sister and I had driven home after Dad arrived for the night shift.

Dad rang at 9 p.m. "...And then she... died...," his voice quavering.

We went back to pick him up, came home and talked for a while, and the next morning I walked around town, calling in to Mum's friends to tell them the news. Then I got the five trains down to New Cross Gate, the loneliest journey I've ever taken. I got back to my flat, dumped my bag and sank into the sofa. My heart hurt and I cried my eyes out.

Next came funeral, probate, wills, sorting things out, and remembrance, bereavement and learning to live with it, submitting to it. But in those few days, I had a gathering sense of what mattered in life, at that moment and beyond – the kind of lucidity that comes in exceptional circumstances:

- Do your best, Kev
- Care for the people you love
- Make the most of what you've got: your life

This chapter is called "To Parents" because I want to say some things about parents and about being a child with troubles, and what I know about that now, because my mum's dying has cemented the meaning of some things that were for a while fluid and uncertain. I don't want to linger on the subject of death and losing a parent, a subject too massive for me to begin understanding, never mind talking about. Instead I want to say things that might help any parent understand when their child seems so beyond help, depressed, anxious and suicidal, because I've been there: stepped toward the brink of the void and then asked for help and care, which my mum and dad gave me.

There is now nothing more I can say to my mum – any more apologies to make or explanations to offer or joys to share – and I was grateful to be able to say what I could in her final days, that fortnight from the phone call to her final breath.

It was quite simple stuff, but it wasn't as I'd imagined it would be: momentous and heavy with poignancy. Cinematic, as deathbed conversations in films are. Instead it was just a chat – simple stuff. We talked things over a bit, then left them there.

One afternoon I sat on the bed with Mum as she typed out a text to a friend, thanking her for being such a good companion over the years. I unfolded the list I'd written and asked if I could ask a few things.

"Are you afraid, Mum?" I asked.

She said no, she wasn't.

Is there something you want?

She said yes. "Peace."

I hugged her and kissed her forehead.

"Do you remember that time I came up and talked to you and Dad and Les, and said I was sorry, Mum?"

"Oh, that was lovely, Kev," she said. "That meant a lot."

Mum smiled.

The amending I talked about a few chapters ago ("Sobriety") is what I was referring to: something that changed things in my family, the dynamic between me as child and Mum and Dad as parents. This is what happened.

In 2015, on the instructions of my sponsor, I'd travelled up to Shropshire in order to say something to them, namely that I was sorry that I'd caused them worry and alarm, even if, in the crisis back in Berlin the year before, I hadn't been in any sense in control of it (by the way, this trip was the first of several missions; "start with the hardest ones", my sponsor had said). But there was more: for years of my being sullen, grouchy or unresponsive, the manner in which by some irresistible inner force I seemed to regress decades when in family company, becoming a moody teenager again (I doubt I'm alone in doing that). It often happened, and just as often I felt guilty and ashamed about it.

So, I'd asked them to sit round the table while I explained myself, and this new way of seeing things that I'd come to learn: *take responsibility, open up, admit the shame.* I said I was sorry, and they took it very well. The rights and wrongs of it mattered less than this gesture of explanation, some humility or contrition, the wanting to make it better: at the very least, addressing that even though I'd been through the thresher, it had hurt them too.

Worry and alarm. No parent likes to see their child in trouble or at risk, whether the child is two years old or 42 years old.

Time brings perspective and this, at least, is clear to me now, another few years on. When you can't explain what's wrong because you don't even know yourself, because it's beyond language and denies all possibility of relating, it has a blast radius. This is a lesson that cuts both ways: for someone suffering it means an explanation to others will help, one day when the time is right. And for the people around that person, maybe this will help explain the way he or she is, how they can seem so blankly unreachable.

I also told my mum and dad that I was sorry that I'd blamed them, as I had – and as, again, children of all ages often do. Never explicitly but inwardly, because this too was the truth of the matter. Feeling acutely pained, I'd long sifted for answers in childhood narratives and memories, among the fears I'd felt: of abandonment, of being unloved or even unlovable. I'd looked at the frictions between me as infant and them as adult – the rows and misunderstandings that are so inevitable a feature of family life – and taken them as the germinations of this "depression" and this "anxiety" I'd known, and then, at times consciously and at other times unknowingly, I'd sometimes played the blame game as a way to mitigate it, conveniencing myself.

But in reflective moments I also knew that my parents had only ever done their best, and done what they could with what they had; brought me up, fed and dressed me, played with me and taught me, loved and disciplined me in their own way, then taken me in and cared for me when I was on my knees at the age of 42. At least a decade older then than they were when I was born.

Across the table that day I had an objective image of my mum and dad: two people, kindly and acceptant, but growing older and more frail, still struggling to understand life, all of which is impossible to see as the child, the one wrapped up with his or her own torments, whether they are psychological, biological, sociological or anything else.

We're supposed to know how life goes and how to live it, even if we don't; when we have no clue whatsoever and we're lost, troubled and confused. And nowhere more do we accept that supposition for truth or fact than with our parents, as they probably did of theirs.

Not so long afterward, one of mine would be fading away as the cancer spread. One evening a month or so before she died, I watched Dad usher Mum out of bed and into the bathroom. She'd become ghostly. She was talkative, putting on a brave face, but inwardly I knew that she wasn't going to make it. And I guess she knew the same.

So I was glad that, a few years before, we'd said these things, in this clumsy family summit I'd arranged. It united us, switched a polarity around, dismantled some unspoken stuff. It rectified something that helped both them and me, it brought us closer, and I was heartened to hear that as she was dying, Mum felt the same way. It made her smile.

The message: if you've got something you want to say to someone you love, do it today. Make the call, find the time. Summon the heart.

If you can.

Love & patience

At the risk of stating the obvious, the dynamic in my family has changed since Mum passed away. Our relating has softened a little, we talk more, things have opened up. I speak to my sister more, and when I'm with her daughter (my niece) we enjoy making gonzo videos together – dancing and cavorting to music – and posting them on Instagram.

Dad comes down to see me a bit more often these days; it's good to see him getting out, and he enjoys the cheap (even free) bus rides. We mooch around south London, or visit a museum up west, and dine on egg, chips and beans in unsensational cafes.

One day last year he wanted to look at the Thames Barrier, so we ventured down to Woolwich Arsenal on the bus and walked westward, back along the river. We talked a lot about Mum and her life, and about the winter when I lived with them both, after returning from Berlin. I was vaguely aware at the time how hard it must have been for them as I skulked around the house, mumbling inarticulately, cramped and uncertain. Either that, or they'd discover me manically sawing up logs in the garden, or questing off into the nearby fields with my waterproofs on.

The worry and alarm.

"Mum and I knew there wasn't much we could help with, about your illness or your situation at the time, Kev," Dad said, as the evening pulled over the Thames. "So we just thought there were two things that mattered: love and patience. We'd love you, and we'd be patient."

The only things they could do, my parents.

The most important things of all.

When over the last few years people have asked me what they can do to help someone suffering – a child or a friend, say – this is the only advice I can offer.

Love and patience.

PART III

MENTAL HEALTH

If you're beginning to feel a bit better, this section
includes some subjects to help you stay that way

CHAPTER 11

PRACTICE

*Why life is a combination of the things that happen to you,
and the things you do every day*

One more guilty secret.

The first job I ever had was washing dishes in a pizza restaurant. I was 16 and ever since then I've had the suspicion that I missed my true vocation as what in French is termed *un plongeur*. My favourite book at the time was George Orwell's *Down And Out In Paris And London*, the account of his expedition into penury as he worked as a dishwasher amid sweat and grime in the bowels of the grand Parisian hotels. No career ladder, perks or benefits, nor any great brainpower needed either, only the daily pattern of soak, scrub, stack and polish, day after day.

It's surely one of the most honest jobs there is, and in times of overwhelm I've daydreamed about an alternative existence as a *plongeur* somewhere in the alleys of Paris, enjoying the fleeting sense of fulfilment while contemplating a tower of squeaky crockery, and with it a certain tragic ambivalence: tomorrow they'll be filthy again, and the world turns once more.

I find something absorbing and perhaps even therapeutic in washing up. Some people do needlecraft, others play Tetris, still others sketch: I like washing up, along with sweeping up, cutting wood, digging the earth, tidying my desk and polishing, fixing and ordering things, from socks to punctures to the books on my shelves. As with walking, manual work takes me out of myself for a moment, liquifies thinking into doing. It reminds me that I'm capable as well as cognitive.

But don't worry: in this chapter I won't suggest you jack your job in to wash dishes for a living (maybe you already wash dishes for a living, in which case: respect). At the same time, I don't mean to romanticize labour or drudge work, and I hope I don't come across as a poverty tourist on leave from my existence as a middle-class professional who makes a living typing words into a keyboard for ten hours a day, often more.

This too can be drudgery, but instead I mean something else. Firstly that, as above, the case for working with your hands is strong if you happen to be doing the parallel graft of dealing with depression and anxiety: doing something manual, mechanical and probably uncreative. And secondly, in recovery (anything you learn to do that helps you feel or function better) there's genuine value in repetition, and I think of this in terms of *practice*: doing something every day that helps you function or feel better.

And throughout the book, we've covered a lot things that, in their own way, might help: it began with the voice and the game of finding words to express how you feel, and moved on to making a habit of regular movement, and developing a mindful attitude to the body. We looked at how learning, listening, sobriety and the elements can play a part, and considered the toxins that can impede growth, from shame to dishonesty to a preoccupation with status. We've gone into subjects that may help summon a clearer outline of the vocational you (the person who's more than their profession) and the relational you (the one who exists in kinship and connections with others). I mentioned at the beginning of this book that it's not uncommon for people who've recovered from crisis to effect a radical turnaround in their lifestyles, so maybe some of this has awoken something similar in you: the urge to pack in your job and pursue an entirely new calling, such as yoga teacher, therapist, wellness app developer, Shaolin monk, full-time artist. Along with *plongeur*, those have all been fantasy alternative careers of mine too.

But still, none of these things is the answer. Instead, the combination of some, many, others or all is the closest we'll come to a solution, along with the dedication to keep repeating the ones that work.

It's often said practice makes perfect, but we're not looking for perfect here, just progress: a one per cent improvement in state or functioning, every day. I mean the modifications you can make to your routine and rituals, and the habits you can start building, starting tomorrow morning. Recall what Bruce the body philosopher said a few chapters ago: "You get better at what you do more of."

That's what this chapter is about, and it begins with something I heard from a couple of guys in Berlin, back in 2013.

Every f***ing day

One dark December night I was lingering in the lobby of a public building in Mitte, not far from the TV Tower, searching for a sign on the door. It was Wednesday, and I was looking for the alcohol recovery meeting. Ascending the second flight of steps, I ran into two middle-aged blokes lounging on a sofa.

Hands immediately outstretched.

"Wassyaname buddy?"

"Kevin."

"*Welcome.*"

I chatted with these guys for a few minutes. They were laconic and placid, and somewhat grizzled. They talked about how long they'd been coming to these meetings – years, between then – and then, in a thick Texan twang, the American guy said, "We're real f***ing alcoholics, man. We have to practise this shit *every day.*"

"Every f***ing day." The Icelandic guy nodded. "No days off."

I wondered what they meant, because I was new to all this and deeply bewildered, but as the meeting began, I quickly found out. For one thing it meant starting the day off correctly: 20 minutes, every morning, meditating and reading, and probably praying too: orienting themselves in the proper direction. Writing inventories of the self-development work they were undertaking. Then, a series of actions and attitudes carried into the day – staying alert to signs of egomania, dishonesty or resentment, for instance (resentment, the blokes explained, was especially poisonous and escalated the likelihood of a relapse. "Resentment is like drinking poison and expecting the other person to die," the Icelandic guy told me. They counselled staying vigilant against it.) And later, as the day drew to a close, another moment of self-reflection, note-making, meditation and prayer. Bed, and then the practice starts again the next morning.

*Every f***ing day.*

This practice they spoke of worked in the sense that neither of them had had a drink or taken a drug for years, obviating the rapid slide into the chaos of inebriation. They talked about how their lives had changed for the better since making a habit of these things, and if sometimes it felt onerous, they knew the commitment was worth it. They shouldered it. Similarly, they talked about how over time all this practice turned into something more substantial: craft, a combination of spiritual rectitude and practical shrewdness that helped them navigate the trouble that life gratuitously dishes out to people whether they're sober, abstinent, using or off their heads: business problems, relationship or family dramas, philosophical quandaries, decisions to be taken.

I admired these blokes, and began to follow their example, doing what was suggested in the book, *Living Sober*, that I'd been given.

Sixty sober days later I realized that the practising itself had become almost automatic: up and out of bed joyously free of a hangover, I'd start the day the way it had been suggested: phone off; a coffee and a notepad; breathing, reading and speaking, with Berlin's fresh winter sun streaming through the windows.

Things began to change; these reflective activities helped and the eternity of the future didn't look so terrifying when I whittled it down to one day at a time. Making a plan for that day and that day only, adding some helpful plug-ins (phone a friend for a chat; make time to walk around the park), and sticking to this principle – every day.

* * *

When enduring a mood disorder it's easy to forget we have choice and some degree of free will: the ability to make a decision and enact it, being proactive (taking the initiative) as well as reactive (responding to events). Decisions and actions repeated day after day build into a continuum, a pattern of progress that endures over time and comes to assume an energy and substance of its own.

On the other hand, it's notoriously difficult, if not impossible, to make decisions that last a year, let alone an entire lifetime (planning, as someone once told me, is a great way of measuring failure). Projects collapse or fall short of expectations not only because life, doing what it wants, gets in the way, but also because we run out of energy or inspiration. We drift off, abandon things. In the face of even the most solemn vows the future remains uncontrollable, bluntly indifferent to our dreams and schemes.

This goes beyond addiction or dependence, of course: it applies generally. Members of the fellowships see recovery as the process of living sober or clean, but if we're to stretch the definition a little, it becomes easy to see that this discipline of daily decision-making and decision-doing is one of the most powerful tools of all, and it maps well onto the recovery from crisis or episodes of depression and anxiety. Developing a daily practice is a way to build positive habits but it's also a way to take the sting out of the immensity of the future. And what is anxiety if not a preoccupation with all the tomorrows? In fact, where practice meets the caprices of fortune, fate, destiny and all the other names we have for "the external world" – this, it seems to me, is precisely what delineates the lives we lead.

The scenario with the two blokes described above happened some months before my crisis moment really struck, but it was in its aftermath when *doing things that help and doing them every day* really began to take on some significance. The principle of practice had stuck with me even when I didn't stick with it. And some time later, in the months and seasons that followed, the portfolio of practices I'd learned began to grow with new ideas and actions I found. Given the nod by those grizzled sages in a room above a school in Berlin, I'd begun to find a path.

When I found myself back in the UK a year later, I picked the practice regime back up again, and starting every day with meditating, reading, praying and writing seemed to assist sanity as well as sobriety. That's when I also noticed the elevation in mood effected by walking, sawing wood and my inept attempts at trikonasana or the sun salutation when I did yoga.

However, what I had to hand wasn't quite enough, so I read further afield, buying wise and helpful books, watching lectures on YouTube and consuming podcasts; and I began to reconnect with friends and contacts in the UK, listening to what they had to say. Maybe I could learn something, I thought. I was receptive – desperately so, in fact – to anything that might help.

More help arrived.

"Find your own pace, and take the time to do it" was something my friend Dawood counselled when on a visit down to London I laid out the debris of my life as I saw it, fretting over the near future. He meant: take it easy, stop chasing. Thing will happen when they need to.

Then there was a line I saw tattooed on someone's arm one evening, which read **"It Is Always Now – You Are Always Here"**, a reminder that while it's all too easy to live in the future with its infinity of What-Ifs?, it's healthier to stay in the present moment.

Meanwhile, **"Stay Teachable"** was what the people in the fellowships kept urging me to do. It made perfect sense once I'd glimpsed the truth of it: there's always more to learn, and we get into trouble the moment we think we know everything there is to know.

And when I was talking to a yoga teacher one day, she offered a further wise observation: **"The best time to plant a tree was twenty years ago. And the second-best time is today."** How true it sounded: regrets hold us in the past, yet every morning brings the chance to start anew.

Perhaps those last two sum up the spirit of practice better than anything else: keep learning, and start applying the learnings today.

These epithets and ideas seemed to be floating in the ether, materializing suddenly like speech bubbles above conversations, graphic and resonant. Notions that can be picked up and enacted, like objects on a sushi restaurant conveyor belt, they belong to no one and everyone at the same time. So I added them to my notebook, reading them over each morning and meditating on them as I walked the streets.

Still, even all this wasn't quite enough. Or rather, eagerly searching for more entries, I began reading further afield and experimenting with physical ideas too: diet hacks, exercise disciplines and bodily techniques to add to the tried and tested routines I already knew well: get into nature, perform the sun salutation, do some shadow-boxing; sit in a chair and scan the body, relaxing each muscle in turn; make a point of going to bed before 10 p.m. And so on. Every f***ing day.

If at times it was tedious or demanding to keep doing the same things again and again, when I lacked energy or simply couldn't be bothered, the overall effect was nevertheless positive and as the months passed I observed a slackening in the tides of anxious thoughts or despairing rumination.

But there was one major downside: prone to being obsessional as I am, I was over-practising. I'd find myself pinging out of bed before the alarm went off and immediately settling myself into a meditation; then I'd urgently rifle through my copy of *Meditations*, looking for a pithy aperçu from Marcus Aurelius to take into the day. Running kit and trainers on, I'd march into the back garden and jog round it ten or twenty times to get the serotonin flowing, adding in some shadow-boxing moves on the side. Then it was back inside to inhale a low-carb, high-protein breakfast before moving on to some sun salutations, an hour of fevered journaling. Meanwhile the pile of logs at the bottom of the garden would be winking at me as if to say, "Well, we're not gonna saw ourselves up, mate." I'd spend afternoons getting stuck in with Dad's bow saw.

As I boot camped myself toward a higher state of transcendent better-ness, my mum looked on, politely mystified.

One morning, panicked by my own zeal for recovery, I rang my friend Jon, bleating about the overwhelm I felt: there just wasn't enough time in the day to get everything done, despite the fact that I was unemployed.

"Kev," said Jon, after a moment. "Pack it in. How about doing one or two of these things every day, rather than trying to do everything at once?"

It made sense. "Find your own pace," Dawood had said. I'd forgotten how doing absolutely nothing – viewing inactivity as an actual thing, a choice – was just as important as doing something. Practising passivity as the natural complement to activity, and doing that every day too because it's amid the sequence of days where change begins to happen.

Here are some of the more simple practices that helped me along the way, and still do.

Fifty breaths: count them in and out

I often found that getting into a meditation was much harder than actually meditating: I'm often too fidgety or distracted. But breathing 50 times and counting the in- and out-breaths is an effective way to enter the state. When we're relaxed we breathe around eight times per minute, so this practice also amounts to a five-minute reset.

Flâneur: go for a walk with no destination. Turn back once you get there.

A way of letting go of the idea of a destination, and to help you get lost in the moment. Most of the walking we do is destined: there's usually an arrival or a goal at the far end of it. Walking in this destination-less way can be disorientating – but that's the point. Allow yourself to get lost in sights and sounds for a while. Give the mind a break from ceaselessly striving.

Smile

Not because, as they say, it will make you happy (this is known as the "facial feedback hypothesis"). But smile because it's more likely to connect you to other people and instigate conversations.

Cultivate patience

It's a virtue, after all. Impossible as it is to imagine any other reality when you're in the bleak winter of a depressive episode, it's a fact that things change, often without our being much involved in the process. Night always turns into day, eventually.

Ask: what's out of balance?

I used to pull a face when people solemnly told me that striving for balance was wise; I'd long thought that life was most interesting at its extremes. These days I see the value in spotting excess and then avoiding it. Change begins with awareness, and recognizing that there's too much of one influence, force or presence in your life is the first step to restoring balance.

Non-attachment: what can you let go of?

One of the central ideas of Buddhism is that attachment causes suffering (loving always entails the risk of heartbreak). This practice isn't to advocate a complete mortification of desire, but instead to become more aware of the things we attach to – objects, outcomes, destinations, dreams and wished-for situations – and gently release ourselves from their grip. It's not easy to do and takes practice – probably a lifetime's worth.

How to stop stopping
(plus, randomizing your recovery)

There's a bit more to say about this Practice idea. Firstly, that the emphasis is on positive doing – building and adding to a helpful routine, tinkering with it – whereas the emphasis in much of the available health advice is on renunciation and denial: don't drink, smoke, take drugs, drive too fast, eat saturated fats, stay up late, sit on the sofa all day, and so on. These all make sense. However, I also found that habits can be changed by adding more of them into the same 24-hour space, and then forcing them to compete. For example, knowing I need to get up early because I've committed to going walking with friends is a great way to stop me staying up too late the night before and fruitlessly pondering the meaning of life.

According to one study by academics at UCL in London, it takes 66 days to build a new habit: just over two months.[17] So, if you're trying to stop some unhealthy habits, one of the fastest ways of doing that is to add in some new and healthier ones.

The second thing to say is that, for me at least, rigidity can instill anxiety. And while the benefit of generating routines doesn't need much more explaining, it's also good to switch things up and surprise yourself. Which is why, one day toward the end of 2015, I took another tack with the expanding library of practices I'd gathered. I went into town and bought a pack of index cards and a set of watercolours, then came home and painted each practice on a card. From then on, I shuffled the pack each morning, picked two cards at random and tried to carry out at least one practice every day. It turned out that often, one was enough – sufficient, at least, to know that I was doing something to energize and accelerate my recovery, while also ensuring that it never became too repetitive. After all, having to decide what to do every morning is tough and sometimes it helps to be told, even when chance itself is the only available authority. When life is random, it makes sense to randomize recovery too, turning it into a game.

In 2017 these index cards turned into something Enver and I published alongside the *Torchlight* book we'd made. They're called "Practice Cards": a pack of 56 playing cards that list all of these things that helped me through the toughest times, and which keep helping me today. From what I've heard from people who use a pack, they help them too.

There are two kinds of card: yellow "Action" cards (suggestions such as performing the sun salutation, shadow-boxing, getting into nature and so on) and blue "Idea" cards: those epithets and ideas harvested from the stock of popular wisdom, along with some consoling thoughts from philosophy, faith and spirituality. There are some general themes within the cards that reflect what we've talked about in previous chapters – ways of connecting with others, methods for reimplanting yourself back in your body, suggestions to develop a practice of self-reflection. And there's one final card with an extra, very important idea: to take a day off from practising. The card shows a slice of pizza, because sometimes spending a day on the sofa is, paradoxically, the way of well-being.

If everything I've said here makes you think that there's isn't a single, ultimate, fail-safe, silver-bullet-style secret method of getting better, a magic solution to all torment and misery, then once again: apologies. There isn't, or at least I haven't found it yet.

The good news is that instead there are hundreds and probably thousands of methods for incremental improvement, and when they're found, configured, arranged and discarded the way they best suit you, then you'll be left with something that can't be bought or found anywhere else, something no one else can tell you: your own practice. Something that will grow and change as you do too. So, find what works for you and keep doing it, every day.

If you've got some practices already, make a note here and add them to your story.

An Idea: _____

_____

_____

_____

An Action: _____

_____

_____

_____

Morning ritual: the basics

Morning rituals are popular these days, with good reason: the first 20 or 30 minutes of the day can offer a moment in which to centre yourself, reflect, make a plan and begin carrying it out, aiming your day in the direction you'd like to see it go. It's probably no coincidence that people with faith, from monks and nuns through to recovering addicts and yoga practitioners, are strict about the first half hour after waking. Don't be put off by the word "ritual": it just means a habit you practise every day, or as often as you're able.

Some elements of a useful morning ritual are described below. These can be adapted or added to suit your own rhythm or taste. However, don't let a failure to achieve the perfect morning ritual every single day turn into another reason to beat yourself up. It's not a competition.

1. **Make your bed.** A useful trick that has helped a lot of people struggling with mental illness. Get up and make your bed, and by the time you get back into it at the end of the day (which could be as little as a few hours later if you're really unwell), at least you'll have achieved one thing. All things considered, a made bed can be a massive achievement.

2. **Meditate.** At its most basic, mindful meditation is non-judgemental moment-to-moment awareness: settling the body, stilling the mind, focusing on the breath as it enters and exits the body, noticing what you're noticing and then letting it pass, seeing thoughts for what they are – just thoughts. Often, it's helpful to have a simple image in your mind: a river flowing past or a hot-air balloon rising into the skies, for example.

   Try counting the breath 50 times, or reading a passage from a book of proverbs, some poetry or a text that says something meaningful to you. Perhaps speak a few words or send up a prayer, devotion, mantra or affirmation. The key thing is to allow the mind to wake up and settle rather than bombarding it with social media, urgent emails and other stimuli. So: avoid your devices for a while.

3. Move. Serotonin is thought to cause the feeling of well-being and moving helps it circulate. Try walking for 15 minutes, or perform a series of stretches or, if you feel dynamic, go for a jog or workout session or do some dancing. Above all, it's important to remind yourself that you are not your thoughts alone: you're a body too.

4. Eat and drink something. But beware strong coffee and tea first thing. Stimulants might put you in a state of alertness (which can also be enjoyable; try as I might, I can't break the habit of an unctuous espresso or five several minutes after waking) but too much can cause anxiety and a boom and bust cycle in mood.

Fat- and protein-based breakfasts (eggs, yoghurt, nuts and so on) have overtaken starchy cereals and pastries in popularity, partly because they don't cause the spike in blood sugar that produces an insulin response that can in turn cause drowsiness.

5. Journaling. What used to be called "keeping a diary". Many people find it helpful to spend some time turning thoughts into text by writing, for example, thoughts and feelings from the day before, visions for the day ahead and dreams from the night in between. This can be useful to look back at from some point in the future, as a way of recording your natural fluctuations in mood. Don't worry about whether the text is spelled correctly or makes any sense. Just allow it to flow out.

6. Ring someone. Just for a chat. Using the voice is a way to remind yourself that you have one, and speaking is a way of entering the world beyond your skin. Nor does it need to be a deep and meaningful interaction. Perhaps call someone and wish them a nice day. They'll appreciate it.

CHAPTER 12

PATIENCE & CHANGE

The final pieces in the mosaic. Plus what story can do for you, and why surrender isn't the end, but the beginning

Chop wood carry water

Today I'm nowhere special, just at my desk shuffling a pack of those Practice Cards, searching for a cue. One card in particular has been winking at me for the past few days, so I stick it on the wall in front of me, in the line of sight. It reads "Chop Wood Carry Water": a saying from Zen Buddhism that I came across a few years ago, probably in an Alan Watts book. In full it reads:

"Before enlightenment, chop wood carry water. After enlightenment, chop wood carry water."

Enlightenment? It's a powerful, cosmic-sounding word but it captures something of the before-and-after curve of the last few years in my life, the winding path from rock bottom to recovery with its sudden breakthroughs and dispiriting setbacks. But what does this saying mean? Simply that on the far side of a big change in life it's important to keep doing the menial and mundane things that keep us grounded. Stock the woodpile, wash the pots, fetch and carry. Stay on top of things, because the work is never done. Life goes on. Get up every day and approach it purposefully.

That's guidance enough, but before I get on with work, I reflect upon where I was when I first heard this phrase. I'd been in France, staying with some friends who'd moved there to open a restaurant. Being penniless at the time, I earned my keep by helping out with the *plonge* (washing dishes), and sawing up wood in the back garden. Some boughs of a huge tree had come down in a gale, so I bought a new blade and got to work, using offcuts to build a den for my friends' daughter. This first visit, it was a year to the day after being hauled up from the pavement and taken to hospital, and I spent quite some time sitting in a plastic chair in the garden, soaked in sweat, noticing something: the gradual return of a neurological glow, my vision clearing, subtle sensations arising.

Since then I've often been back to stay with these friends: holidays from my desk-bound, single-occupancy life, and a chance to reflect on the course of the last few years, this recovery I've been in. There was a basic chronology at the start of this book, but to update it at this end of the tale, here's how it looks:

2013: Blind panic. My coordinates untethering along with a sense deep down that something needed to change in my life, although I didn't know quite what, or how. The clues were all there: problems at work, excesses of hedonism, struggles with relating and the search for meaning.

2014: Began okay, and life was clear, bright and more sober than usual; I was in love (a story for another time). Then out of nowhere: collapse. That day outside that tower block I knew I was done: beaten, licked, on the ropes and at the far edges of whatever agency I had left. The sudden choice: end it all, or ask for help. Back from Berlin to the UK, my possessions shoved into a cellar for storage, then a raw, lonely winter. Walking the streets, teeth clenched, frightened, and consumed by an inner fog.

2015: Tentative beginnings-again. The sun came out as I moved to Bristol, and I began again with the little energy I had, applying myself to getting better. Discovering things, trying new ways to live and develop. The love story from the year before ended, bringing heartbreak. But also, wanting to laugh again. My emotional spectrum began broadening to a wider aperture, colours reappearing in the field of monochrome.

2016: A stabilization in the circumstances of my life (a job and a place to live), as in my mood. Diligently working, studying and scribing. The sine waves of fear and despair lengthening out. They were less intense but nevertheless they were still there, sudden eruptions of dread and periods of blank emptiness. But also I began to feel something else: pops of happiness. Here's how Sigmund Freud defined the term: it "arises from the sudden satisfaction of pent-up needs. By its very nature it can be no more than an episodic phenomenon".[18] Episodic was enough.

2017: Some energy consolidated, and I started speaking more publicly, telling people what I'd told friends and relatives, therapists and mentors: secrets and shames. This new project went very well: for 24 hours I was famed for being depressed, appearing on the cover of a national magazine. Then one of the worst things imaginable happened: my mum died. Life stretched to polar extremes of blessing and blight.

2018: Aftermath. Depressive episodes and bereavement, but practice and industry too. I wrote this book, went running, did the tai chi 24 form, running through steps and strikes. Mornings in the park, afternoons digging the garden. Chop wood, carry water.

2019: Here we are. From bad to worse to better to good to bonkers to this morning. Today.

When I examine this list, some of it looks like the vocation of recovery, dealing with (what we call) mental illness; other elements are merely the events of "life" (heartbreak and bereavement, for instance) and the response they demand from me. But as time passes, they merge into one, the narrow clinical divisions of mental health and illness collapsing still further into each other.

Us, again

Just a few pages left now, and it's also on my mind to ask what, if anything, you've heard in these stories and ideas and whether again you trust my telling of them. We've rattled through a lot, looking at some big subjects, even if we've only really skated the surfaces of learning, body, sobriety, work, nature and so on. There's much more that could be said on each but I hope they've suggested some direction for your path of travel. If you too were at rock bottom or somewhere near, then maybe you're a little elevated now and have found some airspace; maybe you're in motion or movement, equipped at least with something that offers the help you were looking for.

Movement is, I reckon, the soul of recovery: a shift from something to something else. A flux over time that needs one last thing, something that goes above therapy, meds, workouts, list-making, reading, eating, the elements, meditating or anything else we've explored. I mean patience, which is a virtue, but for our purposes is *the* cardinal virtue. Depression and anxiety may seem to bend the laws of time, holding you in a morbid past or accelerating you into a terrifying future. But as that tattoo I mentioned put it, it is always now, and patience – sitting with this painful *now* for as long as it lasts – is what will get you through until everything changes (like trust and acceptance, patience isn't some innate quality doled out haphazardly by the gods, by the way. Instead it's a skill: something that can be learned).

Change it will, and here's where I need to break the promise I made at the start, and repeat: it will change. How can we know? Well, check the weather: it changes. Check your diary: it's no longer last month. Check yourself: you're not who you were at 18, you've grown. The pains you knew then probably aren't the ones you feel today, and the same goes for the joys. Change is the law that's on our side and by synchronizing with it, we can ride along with time.

The chronology above tells me some ways in which I've changed. I never thought I could handle a loved one dying, or stay sober for seasons on end, publish stories that tell the truth as I felt it. And even if I hoped for it, I didn't think I could wake up and simply not be depressed. But that's the way it is today.

Recovery

Recovery is what these last notes are about and we can treat it the way we did some other words, namely "depression" and "anxiety". I mean, in the way we understand it and what it means. Because it too is open to interpretation: there's recovery as anything you learn to do that helps you feel or function better, as we've understood here; recovery as enduring sobriety, as the fellowships see it; there's recovery of the emotions and the nervous system, of desires and drives returning too. The simplest sense of recovery is getting better, improving physically, mentally and spiritually all together, you cohering as a person once again.

What this means in real terms is best posed as a question. How do you know when you're recovered, and how long does it take? The chronology above suggests that it's a matter of years. Bones need six weeks to mend. What about a self?

One answer is simple and perfectly acceptable: you're recovered when you can say, "I'm completely fine, thanks, and I don't need any of this stuff any more. I'm good; I've moved on, it's behind me. The phase is in the past."

The other answer is more substantial and it's what I mean when I say recovery and life have become, for me, the same thing. In this reading, you're never recovered because the adaptations and integrations along the way become the new mode; perhaps even an entirely new way of life.

Phoenix from the flames, the snake shedding its skin, the seven-year life cycle of death and rebirth in human life (this idea is Chinese in origin), or the "spiritual awakenings" we hear about, after which nothing seems the same – there are plenty of dramatic clichés to describe this process, but the truth is that it is something slower and more subtle, almost tectonic, and not always easily explainable nor even identifiable. Doing and seeing things differently, and a change of heart as much as a change of mind.

Perhaps also a change of disposition, and when I think about mine today, I can see a blend of useful flavours in it, the consolations I've learned from the material I've referred to in this book.

I mean that there are elements of:

Existentialist: the ideas we heard from the Parisian philosophers and from Viktor E. Frankl. Life seems to have no intrinsic meaning, so the game is to find your own. The need to do so seems urgent when you're depressed, because depression often results from loss, in this case a loss of meaning – when you can't see "the point". And yes, it's probably best seen as a game instead of a wearisome project of work or study. Games are either won or lost, and the deciding factors are skill and chance. Looked at this way, there is never failure, only learning.

Humanistic: the Carl Rogers stuff. Enter into the lives of others, see things from their point of view and thereby change your own. Interact and empathize. Be there for them, and not merely because it releases you from yourself for a while.

Stoic: from Marcus Aurelius and, in a roundabout way, the teachings of Zen and Tao. Change is the law: everything changes, including you. Hence, again, patience is a virtue. It will change. The block of time you're presently inhabiting will shift, ceding passage to another.

Spiritual, maybe even religious: the stuff I've found in the fellowships. Perspective comes when you set yourself in relation to something massive, or at least bigger than you, bringing the liberation of powerlessness and a relief from the self. The simplest way to effect that is to get involved in group, mission, team, cause, faith or fellowship, and serve it rather than expecting it to serve you.

Mystic: I'm sceptical of ideological or utopian modes of thought these days, nor do I believe that everything can or should be known or answered at the level of rational understanding. Perhaps I sound like a romantic when I say that life isn't a scientific equation to be formulated but a mystery to be embraced, as Madonna sang in "Like A Prayer", which in 1989 was a Number One hit in 20 countries around the world. Mystic Madge knew the score. Let it remain mysterious.

Tragic: in the end, everything ends. It's tough to hear, but it's true. So try to enjoy the path and celebrate the fact that you're on one. I sometimes think that depression is tragedy without the celebration of catharsis, the purging that makes the pain worthwhile.

I'm not saying this is the right way to see the world. It's just the way I see things these days.

Story

There's a useful way of measuring recovery and it's why throughout this book I've hinted at the importance of story, nagging you to note down dreams and moments of change, things you hear as you go through your days, inspiring ideas and pithy observations you've overheard or read in a book, songs to dance to and playlists for varying moods, your gratitude list and practices, your actions and ideas. Here's one last addition, a template to give it some structure:

How did it start?

When did it change?

What happened next?

What does it mean?

In its simplest sense storytelling means speaking, and as I hope is plain by now, speaking about a problem is the first step in dealing with it. This has done a lot for me, and I reckon it can for anyone, because while labels only take you so far, providing a frame of reference, a story will take you further. A label such as "depression" holds you in the static paradigm of diagnosis, but a story is a dynamic structure: it's a chronicle, the report of change over time, and it's valuable because humans are dynamic too. Once more, this is what Carl Rogers talked about with his idea of "becoming".

A story helps you notice how you've adapted and reacted, tracking the motion of ill to well, better to worse and back again, because the fact is that the self changes too, especially in the earthquake of a crisis, breakdown or burnout. Therapy, as my therapist said, is like a coil but so is living: we may be going around in circles but we're moving forward. So, if recovery is change from one state or perspective to another, story is what records the change, whether it is made in writing, speaking or any other medium that facilitates it: dancing or tai chi, say.

But story can also animate that change, giving it energy and form. The psychotherapist Adam Phillips once wrote about "the talent for transforming madness into something other than itself, of making terror comforting. Sanity is this talent for not letting whatever frightens us about ourselves destroy our pleasure for life; and this... is essentially a linguistic talent."[19] Words and stories can set us apart from the things that terrorize us and when it's eventually possible to see recovery as a creative process as well as a biological, psychological or clinical one, then it may become the most creative thing you ever do. Showing it to others will probably help them too, letting them know they're far from alone, and that the ghosts haunting them have been known before.

The last word

One final yarn from this story that ends where it began, in Berlin.

I was over there again recently, to speak at a conference organized by a friend, Jacob, and this time found myself sat in a circle of chairs with 20 or so others, in a renovated factory building. Sunshine was refracting through the big windows that morning, and the focus of discussion was well-being in the music business – something I knew literally nothing about – and there were presentations on mindfulness, Greek philosophy and the elusive work–life balance.

Directly opposite me in the speaker's chair was a woman of, I guessed, about my age, and she was talking about the burnout she'd had – the second, in fact – while working in the music industry. Listening to her I found myself nodding in agreement, recognizing passages from her story that matched my own with an uncanny fidelity: the feeling of being unable to cope; the course of events when she began to accept help from doctors, therapists, family and friends; and how she lives life now: calmly and wisely, looking after her family, working when she's able or feels like it. After she'd finished I felt the urge to pipe up, and share something back as the group listened.

"There's so much I recognize from what you've said, I can hardly believe it," I said. "I mean, I've been there too – on the floor. At rock bottom. Not far from here, in fact... just over by Alexanderplatz, a few years ago."

The silver eyeball of the TV Tower was watching us through the window.

After the session ended she and I chatted and exchanged email addresses. We didn't say much, perhaps because we didn't need to: it was as if there was some channel of understanding between us, a shared familiarity with the depths of crisis. The bleak flatness when none of your faculties – speaking, thinking, moving, liking – work anymore. The surging dread upon waking, and the locked-in hopelessness throughout the day.

People who've been in these states often return from them deeply changed, I've noticed. Not transformed into some finger-snapping, Californian-style Positive-Mental-Attitude optimist, but something else. I could intuit it in this person and I had a sense that somewhere along the path we'd both been walking, she'd lost some shroud of unnecessary shame. There's an upside to these experiences, though it's impossible to imagine at the time.

People live through the worst of these episodes and often go on to great things, but the definition of "great" has changed: many lead very ordinary, unsensational lives, often built on an awareness that the crisis could happen again. Lives that may seem a few rungs further down the aspirational ladder but which, from the vantage point of rock bottom, are nevertheless miraculous. Once they've stopped striving for perfection, constant stimulation and total fulfilment, these people want their lives only to be liveable and peaceful, and maybe mean a little, to themselves and a few others.

The pattern of my own episodes tells me I'll probably never be in the clear or fully "cured", and I'll need to stay alert to oncoming lows, dealing with them as and when they arrive. Doing so involves as much passivity as effort. I say that because we often hear talk of celebrities "battling" mental illness, as if they're on a crusade of grimly tenacious effort with the ultimate goal of conquering it once and for all, completely and forever. While the activity of recovery often resembles something like asymmetric warfare – a daily guerrilla campaign against an unpredictable, shape-shifting enemy – it's also true that it only really begins with something antithetical to will and effort.

I mean a surrender to need, and asking for help. A submission to the enveloping fog as it passes over and then, later on, a further submission to change itself, and letting these changes change you. Letting your story write itself, and go where it will.

Still, anxieties are like barnacles: they stick around.

After lunch I said goodbye to Jacob and the other participants and, needing to stretch my legs, I began walking down Karl-Marx-Allee, the wide boulevard that travels east from the TV Tower. This was my running track when I lived in Berlin, and in the evenings I often jogged the five kilometres down to Frankfurter Tor and back, sprinting the last few hundred metres, finishing spent and emptied under the sun and sometimes the snow.

Somewhere around Strausberger Platz I stopped to rest on a bench for a while, looking at Facebook and Instagram. The usual promises of transformation: an advert for a 21-day yoga body shred, another how-to video on getting a six-pack. Banal wellness memes and lists of things I ought to do, overcome and go beyond and so through force of will, belief or exertion attain some kind of superhuman perfection.

Need to unfollow a few of these accounts, I thought.

I got up and strolled on, then caught sight of my reflection in the window.

Yep: still ugly… shorter than I'd like to be, balder than ever. Laughter lines deeper, my features slipping south.

I squared up to the image, scrutinized it a bit longer and then winked.

It's fine. I'm okay. Everything's cool. No need to try so hard.

It was early evening by the time I got back to my digs, and I wrote down a to-do list for the next day. Emailing the lady in the speaker's chair was the first thing, to express how much I enjoyed meeting her. I also wanted to pass on something that someone once said to me, with a smile on his face – something I'd like to pass on to you too:

I wish you a long recovery.

GRATITUDE

How it works and why it's healthy to practise it

Tony Robbins once pointed out that it's impossible to be angry if you're grateful. It's a useful idea for sure. Left unchecked, anger burns people up, while gratitude – an awareness of what you're thankful for – douses the flames.

Practising gratitude can do something else. It's a cleanser, sloughing off ill-will, irritation and malice, and it's a reminder that your life might not be quite so bleak as it appears. The simplest way of doing it is by making lists of the things you're grateful for, or even more simply the things you've got, switching attention from what you haven't got. What's also called *counting your blessings*.

I reflect on that this morning, and I begin writing today's list:

- The bed I sleep in with a roof above it.
- The desk I bought in Berlin and hauled back to the UK, which I'm sat at now.
- Really obvious stuff: health, five functioning senses, running water, safety, money enough to pay the rent, sausage and chips for dinner.
- This day.
- Numbers: the digits of friends and relatives on the other end of a line, available even if they're not present.
- These legs that have walked me far and wide, the arms that I've wrapped around others as others wrapped theirs around me.
- The fingers that typed out these thoughts.
- That one doesn't need permission to say these things.
- For teachability too. Stories don't end; all closure is temporary.
- For truly awful weather that makes me appreciate the coming of sun and warm winds.

– Thankfulness also for the tough times I've known with despair, depression, fear and crisis, heartbreak and disappointment and the good times that follow them: a run down Karl-Marx-Allee, a walk around the park, a laugh with friends, heart emojis incoming on WhatsApp.

It's easy to forget these things, but this is what abundance looks like when I stop taking things for granted. It lifts me by millimetres, which is sometimes all I need.

* * *

While we're on the subject of gratitude, here seems like the right place to acknowledge the people without whom this book wouldn't have been possible. I'm grateful to those who gave their time and expertise to put muscle on the bones of these stories, experts in their field who also see wisely what lies beyond them: Dr Ian Drever and Dr Will Napier, Esher Groves; Dr Luke Sullivan, Men's Minds Matter; Dr Jane McNeill; Stacy Thomson, Performance Club; Rose Scanlon-Jones, Sanctus; Dawood Gustave and Adam Papaphilippopoulos, Reluctantly Brave; Bruce Butler, Motus Strength; Amy Orben, University of Oxford; Dr Ben Sessa, Mandala Therapy; Nadia Gilani; Jamie Richards; Georgie Mack, Minds@Work.

Writing, speaking and publishing about these subjects goes a bit further back in time, but none of it would have gone beyond the narrow sphere of my own thoughts without (especially and tirelessly) Enver Hadzijaj, Emma Warren and Paul Kellett Van Leer; plus Zaren Courtenay, Laura Clark, Sam Blunden and Callum Jefferies. Meanwhile this book arose from a conversation with my editor, Tara O'Sullivan, and wouldn't exist without her, along with her colleagues Isabel Gonzalez-Prendergast, Joanna Copestick, Caroline Alberti, Karen Baker, Meg Brown, Kari Brownlie and Paul Palmer-Edwards.

The helping society: since the day I folded in Berlin a lot of people have helped me in ways they may never be aware of, freely and without thought of recompense. When I pause to enumerate them, among the things they gave me have been: time, attention, listening, fun, care, jobs, lifts, favours, money, occupation, advice, skills, guidance, something to eat, drink, watch, read and think about, somewhere to sleep or rest.

So I'm grateful to: Sean Pillot De Chenecy, Amy Binding, Kati Krause, Nauva Nauva, Margarita MK, Lorena Maza, Paul Snowden, Dr Jeni Fulton, Kai Kirchhoff, Ana Lessing, Grashina Gabelmann, Kai Schaechtele, Melanie Constein, Joerg Koch, Josie Thaddeus-Johns, Paul Sullivan, Gabriele Gollwitzer, Marcel Nawrath, Quynh Tran, Peter Lyle, Warren Jackson, Mark Hooper, Jack Boulter and Deborah Fitzgerald, Simon and Emily Das, Matthew Kershaw and family, Alice Fisher, Johnny Davis, Alex Bilmes, Barney Calman, Charlotte Hillenbrand, Sam Small, Vivienne Berryman, Hannah Tyson, Susan Lin, Peter Parkes, Geoff MacDonald, Melissa Ramos, Liz Helman, Rubens Filho and Abracademy, Andrew Diprose, Bruce Sandell, Jo Watkins, Alfred Rinaldi, Jessica Reitz, Jeremy Leslie, Leigh Bentley, Alise Avota, Chris Gameson, Alice Taylor, Neil Boorman, Clare Reddington, David and Karol Wilson, Hannah Anketell, Lauren Cochrane, Joanna Boffey and Liam Murdoch, Lucy Cook, Layla Sargent, Simmy Richman, Pauline Rhodes, Rob Stephenson, Lucy Oliver, Steve Beale, Danny Flower, Will de Groot, Anne Baerwald, Jacob Bilabel, Maïa Beyrouti, Joy Yoon, Simon Wainwright, Emma Allen, and Tim Pare and family.

For wise counsel: Andrew Sadler, David Baker, Andrew Hobbs, Mark James, Sharmaine Lovegrove and Vanessa Remoquillo.

For the *mousse de canard:* Søren, Mel, Grethe, Nora, Fred and Caro.

For fellowship: John F, Jo C, Dave and the Telegraph Hill Mob.

For firegazing: Johnny Denton, Greg Parker, Ian Danby, David Pearson, John Atkinson and Stu Le Fevre.

As the day comes to an end I think of my family: Dad, Lesley, Andrew and Iona.

In the end: Marion Wilson Braddock (1940–2017), who taught me to read and write, showed me what kindness and love mean.

Rest in peace Ma.

Suggested Further Reading

Some books that have, in one way or another, helped me understand life and the changes we go through as we live

Psychology & philosophy

Marcus Aurelius – *Meditations*
Sarah Bakewell – *At The Existentialist Café*
Martin Buber – *I And Thou*
Anthony De Mello – *Awareness*
Viktor E. Frankl – *Man's Search For Meaning*
Sigmund Freud – *Civilisation And Its Discontents*
Sigmund Freud – *The Interpretation Of Dreams*
John N. Gray – *Straw Dogs*
Søren Kierkegaard – *Fear and Trembling*
Leonard Koren – *Wabi-Sabi For Artists, Designers, Poets and Philosophers*
R.D. Laing – *The Divided Self*
Adam Phillips – *Going Sane*
John Powell – *Why Am I Afraid To Tell You Who I Am?*
Carl Rogers – *On Becoming A Person*
Seneca – *On The Shortness Of Life*
Dr Michael Sinclair & Dr Matthew Beadman – *The Little ACT Workbook*
Nassim Nicholas Taleb – *Antifragile*
Irvin D. Yalom – *Love's Executioner*
Bessel van der Kolk – *The Body Keeps the Score*
Dr Gabor Maté – *In the Realm of Hungry Ghosts*
Darian Leader – *The New Black*
Dr Tim Cantopher – *Depressive Illness, the Curse of the Strong*

Gender

Robert Bly – *Iron John*
Robert A. Johnson – *The Fisher King and The Handless Maiden*
Dan Millman – *The Way Of The Peaceful Warrior*
Naomi Wolf – *The Beauty Myth*

Faith & spirituality

Alcoholics Anonymous – *The Big Book*
Alcoholics Anonymous – *Living Sober*
Steve Hagen – *Buddhism Plain and Simple*
Eugen Herrigel – *Zen In The Art Of Archery*
William James – *The Varieties Of Religious Experience*
Lao-Tzu – *Tao Te Ching*
Deng Ming-Dao – *365 Tao: Daily Meditations*
Alan Watts – *The Book: The Taboo On Knowing Who You Are*
Alan Watts – *The Way of Zen*
The Holy Bible

Narrative

Vincent Deary – *How We Are*
Paul Farley and Michael Symmons Roberts – *Edgelands*
James Frey – *A Million Little Pieces*
James Frey – *My Friend Leonard*
Denis Johnson – *Jesus' Son*
Amy Liptrot – *The Outrun*
Haruki Murakami – *What I Talk About When I Talk About Running*
William Styron – *Darkness Visible*

**To find out more about the Torchlight System, visit www.torchlightsystem.com
or follow @torchlight_system on Instagram.**

Notes

1. https://www.ons.gov.uk/peoplepopulationandcommunity/
    birthsdeathsandmarriages/deaths/bulletins/suicidesintheunited
    kingdom/2017registrations#suicides-in-the-uk
2. *The Economist*, 24 November 2018
3. https://www.theguardian.com/society/2018/aug/06/hospital-
    admissions-for-teenage-girls-who-self-harm-nearly-double
4. https://www.theatlantic.com/business/archive/2017/08/lawrence-
    lessig-aaron-swartz/537693
5. Mental Health Foundation: London, 2016
6. https://www.ncbi.nlm.nih.gov/pubmed/9560163
7. Dr Tim Cantopher, *Depressive Illness: The Curse of the Strong*,
    pamphlet accompanying book of the same name, Sheldon Press, 2003
8. Marcus Aurelius, *Meditations*, translated by Maxwell Staniforth,
    Penguin Books 2004, London.
9. Carl Rogers, *On Becoming A Person*, Constable, London, 2004
10. *Work: How to Find Joy and Meaning in Each Hour of the Day* (2012) by
    Thich Nhat Hanh with permission of Parallax Press, Berkeley,
    California, www.parallax.org
11. Sigmund Freud, *Civilisation and Its Discontents*, Penguin Classics,
    London, 2002
12. https://www.theguardian.com/society/2018/oct/10/young-people-
    drinking-alcohol-study-england
13. https://www.bbc.co.uk/news/health-45487187
14. http://citymha.org.uk/wp-content/uploads/2017/11/MH-Inside-our-
    City-Workplaces-Report-Nov.17.pdf
15. https://assets.publishing.service.gov.uk/government/uploads/system/
    uploads/attachment_data/file/658145/thriving-at-work-stevenson-
    farmer-review.pdf
16. https://www.ons.gov.uk/peoplepopulationandcommunity/
    birthsdeathsandmarriages/deaths/articles/suicidebyoccupation/
    england2011to2015#main-points
17. https://www.ucl.ac.uk/news/2009/aug/how-long-does-it-take-form-habit
18. Sigmund Freud, *Civilisation and its Discontents*, Penguin Classics,
    London, 2002
19. Adam Phillips, *Going Sane*, Penguin, London, 2006